Feeling The Call: Therapeutic Uses of Traditional West-African Drumming

By Signe M. Kastberg PhD LMHC

Cover design by Chloe K. Bogden

Feeling The Call:

Therapeutic Uses of
Traditional West-African Drumming

ISBN-13: 978-1722073565

ISBN-10: 172207356X

CreateSpace Independent Publishing Platform

Table of Contents

Acknowledgements

I want to thank my most important African drumming teachers, starting in Ithaca, NY, with Maurice Haltom and Edward Biko Smith, both of whom shared joyfulness and much laughter as my children and I were introduced to traditional West-African drumming and dancing. My most profound gratitude goes to Khalid Abdul N'Faly Saleem, Music Director for the Sankofa African drumming and dance ensemble at the SUNY College at Brockport, NY. Khalid demonstrated the combined power of gentleness and fierce drumming while simultaneously building community through constant encouragement and engagement with both people and process.   A few other teachers with whom I took class or played for dancers, and who contributed to my growth and understanding are: M'bemba Bangoura, Biboti, Mangue Sylla, Bernard Woma, Michael Markus, and so many more.

Three people who contributed significantly to enhancements in this final manuscript through suggested edits, corrections, and gentle redirection are: fellow drummer Marcia E. Vanderlee, M.S. B.S., Certified Therapeutic Recreation Specialist ; visual neuroscientist and super salsa dancer Russell David Hamer, Ph.D., Affiliate Research Professor at the Department of Psychology, Florida Atlantic University, and Professor Visitante Especial, Departamento de Psicologia Experimental, Instituto de Psicologia at the Universidade de São Paulo, Brasil, and formerly Scientist at the Smith-Kettlewell Eye Research Institute; and one of my original African drumming teachers, Edward Biko Smith. Their time and patience are greatly appreciated.

To the hundreds of clients who have trusted me with their life stories, and their hands, I am privileged to have worked with you. And to the many fellow drummers and dancers who formed a community of meaning that supported and encouraged me and each other, I thank you!

CHAPTER 1

"In the beginning was noise. And noise begat rhythm. And rhythm begat everything else. This is the kind of cosmology a drummer can live with." ~ Mickey Hart, *Planet Drum* (1991, p. 12)

Introduction: The Call

Traditional West-African drumming begins with "the call," a rhythmic signal that we are about to begin, played by the lead drummer of the group. The musical call-and-response pattern originated in Africa (Nketia, 2005), and traces of that original ritual are evident in many American Methodist churches; when the preacher says, "Can I get an A-men," the parishioners respond quickly with "Amen!" In writing about The Call, master drummer Sule Greg Wilson says, "Music is sacred. It is an integral part of the way of life of many traditional cultures throughout the world; it is the invocation of vital energies that ensure a community's survival. Music helps maintain harmony in and with both the visible and invisible world" (Wilson, 1992, p. xiii).

So here I am giving you the call; I invite you to join with me on a collaborative journey of exploration regarding therapeutic uses of traditional West-African drumming.

In Africa, music is important only in relation to the context in which it is played. The music is used to accentuate certain aspects of the event or ritual, to interact with it as a supporting ensemble. If you ask an African how s/he liked the music, s/he might respond in a way that covers the entire social occasion in which the music was played. John Miller Chernoff, a drummer and researcher at Trinity College in Ghana, says that the music may change as the event unfolds, in response to what is happening (1979, p. 67). In short, music is both very context-dependent in this tradition and always a group activity. The musical experience is a community-wide construction. Kalani and Camara (2006) state that there is a traditional rhythm and dance for virtually every life event. Thus, every person in West Africa has the experience of a musical "soundtrack of your life" (p. 20). This allows you to learn not only about yourself, but about the people around you; it is interactive and pervasive.

"Music is essential to life in Africa because Africans use music to mediate their involvement within a community, and a good musical performance reveals their orientation toward this crucial concern" (Chernoff, 1979, p 154). People reveal their opinion and their aesthetic through their participation in the community: if the music is good, the dancing and singing will show it through style and involvement; if it is disappointing; the participants will do what they can to correct it or encourage correction of it. The value of the musical experience is in the participation, and this is reflective of an ethic of interdependency, collaboration, and cooperation within the entire community.

Slaves brought to the US were not allowed to keep their drums; in fact, witness this proclamation from the 1700s:

> "It is absolutely necessary to the safety of this Province, that all due care be taken to restrain Negroes from using or keeping of drums, which may call together or give sign or notice to one another of their wicked designs and purposes."
> — Slave Code of South Carolina, Article 36 (1740)." (Zhao, 2014)

Despite the denial of a mode of expression central to slaves' heritage, their connection to drumming and religious ritual via drumming emerged in a new and powerful way: the blues, jazz, rock and roll (Hart, 1990 p. 210). When we say that African-American music essentially evolved from the music brought by African slaves in the US, we mistakenly frame each tradition as singular. In fact, Africa had/has a multiplicity of musical traditions; thus, many sources contributed to the development of a variety of music and dance forms in the US (Hood, M., in Jackson, ed., 1985). Although multiple forms of drumming will be mentioned here, my focus is on traditional West-African drumming; ie, those songs and meanings originating in countries such as Guinea, Senegal, Mali, Ivory Coast, and Ghana.

"Africans rely on music to build a context for community action" (Chernoff, 1979, p. 161) where participation (musician, dancer) is considered a contribution to the life of the community and to deepening interpersonal connections. The group works together to bring order and stability in a complex world characterized by conflict and opposition. Africans are often flexible in dealing with a complex and sometimes chaotic world, and in fact, in many African languages the word for "guest" is the same as for "stranger".

I began using drumming with clients, and with students, about 12 years ago. As a licensed mental health counselor, I am well-versed in "talk therapy" but alternative methods of reaching clients and encouraging self-expression have been expanding and gaining credence. My own experience learning to drum and becoming enamored with the culture, history, and performance of traditional West-African drumming led me to directly experience and understand the health benefits. We will be exploring the specific health benefits of drumming in a later section.

Music in general, and as therapeutic intervention

Why do humans enjoy music? In a delightful book entitled *Musicophilia*, Oliver Sacks (2007) explored this question. Sacks was a neurologist. While much of our human interaction has a purposeful evolutionary role, music lies outside that realm. Even Darwin was puzzled, as he wrote in *The Descent of Man* (1859): "As neither the enjoyment nor the capacity of producing musical notes are faculties of the least use to man...they must be ranked among the most mysterious with which he is endowed" (cited in Sacks, 2007, p. x). Renowned evolutionary biologist Stephen Jay Gould spoke of music as a non-adaptive change in the human species; that is, an adaptation that has no role in our survival (cited in Sacks, 2007, p. xi). However, Sacks calls us a "musical species" in that we use various components of our complex neural circuitry to perceive music; we appreciate its structure, sometimes use our muscles to echo the timing of the musical narrative, and we often respond with deep emotion (xii).

For many of us, the experience of music is profound. Schopenhauer, a 19th-century philosopher, wrote, "[Music] reproduces all the emotions of our innermost being, but entirely without reality and remote from its pain…Music expresses only the quintessence of life and of its events" (Sacks, 2007, p. xii). Music can calm us, animate us, comfort us, thrill us, or serve to organize and synchronize us at work or play. Music need not even actually be present for us to feel its effects, as we can imagine music. It has powerful therapeutic potential, perhaps particularly for those who do not respond to other therapeutic interventions.

We should not assume, however, that music has therapeutic value for all people. Indeed, Sacks (2007) found that in talking with Temple Grandin about music, while she appreciated the "ingenious" nature of Bach, it stirred no feeling in her. Grandin has Asperger's disorder (on the autism spectrum), and for some with this disorder, the amygdala (part of the limbic system) is poorly developed. Grandin could not state that she "enjoyed" music; only that she appreciated the structure of more intricate compositions. For many others with autism spectrum disorders, music is an effective way to promote interaction, especially with some non-verbal clients who otherwise may be difficult to reach through conventional therapy (Sacks, 2007).

Conversely, at least one of Freud's biographers saw his reported avoidance of music as defensive; Theodor Reik, in *The Haunting Melody,* wrote that Freud protected his ability to analyze and reason without emotions clouding his perception. "He developed an increasing reluctance to surrendering to the dark power of music. Such an avoidance of the emotional effect of melodies can sometimes be seen in people who feel endangered by the intensity of their feelings" (as cited in Sacks, 2007, p. 322). To illustrate the evocative nature of music in an extreme degree, one need only recall photos of throngs of the Beatles' fans, or Elvis Presley's fans, or any celebrity rock star today, in which the audience are in a swoon, or in tears, or screaming in excitement, as they hear their idols play.

It has been suggested that the majority of people in the US have, at some point, been told that they lack musicality. For example, perhaps a parent told a child "you can't carry a tune in a bushel basket." (Disclosure: that was my mother, to me.) Perhaps a youth was told they didn't have rhythm, or their tone was sharp, or flat. Gender bias is sometimes present; more than one girl who asked to play percussion instruments was denied her choice. Music teachers in elementary school play a powerful role as children internalize the opinions of authority figures. Thus, many persons silence themselves musically and avoid attempting to sing (except in the privacy of their car or shower) or learn an instrument. Part of what I do is counter this past negative messaging and encourage my clients to try traditional West-African drumming, and praise them for their efforts.

Music therapy is practiced in some form in most states in the US. In some states, a particular license is required to practice as a music therapist; preparation for licensure requires significant coursework, supervised practice, and examination. For those who are interested, each state's licensure regulations are available on line; there is also credentialing information through professional organizations such as the American Music Therapy Association [see references for website].

"Music therapy studies have shown that rhythm directly affects the psyche. For centuries, shamans have known the spiritual significance and used the healing effects of rhythm. Whoever hears or plays a rhythm changes. This can be measured medically by breath frequency, muscle tone, and the concentration of oxygen in the blood" (Billmeier & Keita 1999, p. 11). More on biological outcomes will be covered in Chapter 4.

"Talk Therapy" is a mode that requires a client able to articulate his/her thoughts and emotions to a therapist who is able to hear and interpret those thoughts and feelings. Some populations are less amenable to talk therapy. Among those for whom alternative methods are desirable are children, persons with certain kinds of disorders, and the elderly. Why? Children are restricted by their vocabulary, and many children lack a "feeling" vocabulary beyond mad-sad-glad-bad. Parents of young children are familiar with the claim, "my tummy hurts," which is often a sign of anxiety or depression rather than a physical illness. Elderly clients with memory deficits, even in the case of dementia disorders such as Alzheimer's Disease, often respond positively to music from their youth, prompting recollections of an earlier time and propelling verbalization. Persons with anxiety and depression may respond well to music therapy after they have articulated their thoughts and feelings but remain "stuck" or blocked in their therapeutic progress.

Why this is *not* about Drum Circles

> "Each performance demands a special attitude, combining
> both discipline and freedom. …the organization of the many
> rhythms imposes restrictions on expression. The old men
> demonstrate the best musical style because they are able to
> let the other parts speak, to build and control a more forceful
> and organized expression. They know how to be free
> without dominating or ignoring the other rhythms, and they
> use their insight to open the rhythmic relationships to
> participation and communication. They demonstrate
> character by knowing the boundaries of participation…"
> (Chernoff, 1979, p. 166)

Aristotle said, "Through discipline comes freedom." My philosophy
in teaching clients traditional West-African drumming echoes
Aristotle: I tell my clients, "With discipline comes freedom." A
prima ballerina doesn't demonstrate excellence on stage after one
week of lessons. A successful artist doesn't fling paint on canvas.
An *haute couture* fashion designer doesn't wad up bunches of fabric
on a model and say *Voila*! Each of these endeavors requires patient
and focused attention to developing skills and techniques. The
foundation of such dedicated development becomes a platform for
showcasing artistry and originality. Discipline is not a feature of
drum circles.

I used to take ballroom dance classes from an Argentinian teacher
named Martin`. Dance progresses from basic steps to more
advanced steps and more advanced versions of those steps. As I
struggled to "do the steps" and to transition to the more advanced
versions, Martin` told me, "How you're doing it [the basic steps] is
not wrong, but *this* [the advanced version] is *better*." The same is
true of the difference between drum circles (very basic, no technique
or finesse required) and traditional West-African drumming
(contextual, polyrhythmic, imbued with meaning). Drum circles are
not wrong or bad; traditional West-African drumming is simply a
richer version with an abundant environment for creating and
exploring various meanings. These meanings will be discussed later
in the book.

According to Chernoff (1979), one of the worst things you can say about a drummer in Ghana is that he plays "by heart". Such an individual acts at random; his expressions are rough and without purpose. In this case, these terms mean that the person is unconcerned for the meaningfulness of his actions, lacks a sense of proportion in self-awareness, and lacks thoughtfulness in self-expression. Random behavior is the exact antithesis of the synchronistic reflective, interdependent musician (Chernoff, 1979, p 166-7).

The self-expression of a drum circle is often random and episodic, lacking the structure and contextual meaning of traditional West-African drumming. Having participated in both venues over a couple of decades, below I have elucidated my understanding of the key differences between the drum circle approach, and traditional West-African drumming.

Traditional West-African	Drum Circle
Commitment	Open, no commitment
Focused	Unfocused
Culturally contextual	A-cultural
Structured	Flexible
Community	Temporary community
Purposeful	Variable/random
Other-focused	Self-focused
Interdependent	Independent
Disciplined	Undisciplined

I'll explain each of these elements. First, the commitment in a traditional West-African drumming group is an allegiance to the members of your group, and respect for the master drummer.

Because the intention is playing for the enjoyment of others (dancers, community), you don't stop playing your part until the song is done. In a drum circle you come and go as the mood moves you or as is convenient. You can stop playing at any time. The traditional West-African drummers are focused because each person plays a part –ie, an assigned rhythm—that is essential to the overall musicality of the particular song being played. The musicians are keyed into each other and the rhythm will ebb and flow. Listening is key to playing well together. In the drum circle there is a lack of focus on the song, because by definition there is no song; simply, the ambient rhythm being invented in the moment has no beginning and no defined end.

Traditional West-African drumming is richly contextual. Songs have meanings typically based on life roles, life transitions, and the natural world (Billmeier & Keita, 1999). The music is based on tradition and history, as are the instruments. The dancers' movements are likewise based on meaningful signifiers, such as honoring the earth or the sun. Drum circles have no cultural context; any instrument can be played, including vocalizations, and have no inherent meaning. Body movement may include a wide array of gestures and I have seen more than a few intoxicated people wander into the drum circle and "perform" for those present. Anything goes: fire twirlers, hula hoops, glow sticks, bongos, congas, guitars, and more.

Traditional West-African drumming is structured. Most songs are polyrhythmic, with mutiple djembe parts. The master drummer usually invites individuals to play those parts such that all parts are covered. Traditionally, you play your part continuously once the master plays the call. In a drum circle, flexibility is the foundation of the event. You can play anything you wish, or nothing at all.

The true purpose of traditional West-African drumming is to reinforce the importance of a shared sense of community. Drummers support each other, and the dancers, in order to bring joy and participation to the audience. Experienced drummers mentor less-proficient rookies. There is an attitude of respect and unity. In a drum circle, since individual freedom of expression is a focus, the sense of community is temporary and time-limited. Anyone can come, anyone can leave; the boundaries are permeable if not non-existent and therefore no commitment is necessary. In the drum circle venue, people are often friendly, but active mentoring is rare, leaving new musicians somewhat lost and without a sense of meaningful participation.

Traditional West-African drumming is purposeful. Drummers don't play for themselves, although that is a nice side benefit; they play for dancers and for the community. A community with a cultural and historical context is reinforced through playing meaningful songs. Drum circles are highly variable in format and content; it is never the same twice, as people come and go, instruments are widely varied from one event to the next, and the songs are invented each time.

As noted above, the traditional West-African drumming is other-focused, playing for others' enjoyment and to reinforce the connections within a community. This is reflective of collectivistic cultures where what's best for the community comes first; self-interest is secondary to group continuity. Drum circles exist for individual pleasure and reinforce Western ideals of individualism.

Traditional West-African drumming is interdependent. If only one person is playing, they can only play one part, and so the song is not as originally conceptualized. The various parts to each polyrhythmic song are intertwined to create a coherent whole. The drum circle participants are completely independent as there is no intent to assign meaning to the sounds that are created. The production of harmonious sounds in the drum circle is a happy accident.

Traditional West-African drumming is a disciplined art. As noted above, the master drummer is one who has perfected his/her technique and developed a high level of skill on his/her instrument. Other drummers work to develop their skills to add to the enjoyment of dancers and others. Drum circles are inherently flexible group events with no pretense at discipline; it would be antithetical to the nature of this activity. As in my previous example of ballroom dance, shuffling your feet and walking around the floor is not "dancing"; many traditional West-African drummers similarly see drum circles as not "drumming" at all.

As we get into the therapeutic applications of traditional West-African drumming, you will see how each of the attributes of traditional West-African drumming contribute to personal growth and development in clients. I'm not suggesting that drum circles cannot be therapeutic; both anecdotal and scientific evidence suggest that they can be healing for participants, both emotionally and physiologically. Much of the existing research, to be discussed in chapter 4, is specifically due to facilitated drum circles. Expert facilitation is a key factor that can give a drum circle momentum and flow (Stevens 2003), but many recreational drum circles lack this feature and are leaderless. We shall see how these essential differences may be particularly valuable for certain populations.

My goals and agenda

My overarching goal is to change the world, but I've been finding that difficult to do alone. I suspect we will have better luck if we attempt this together. As a therapist and a continuous observer of human behavior, I see an increasing sense of disconnection experienced by individuals, even when surrounded by throngs of people. In his book *Bowling Alone* (2000), Robert Putnam details the progression of this phenomenon over decades. We have become a nation of loners, yet the very nature of our species is to yearn for connection. I'm not talking about the connections that come with counting how many Facebook friends you have, or how many LinkedIn followers, or who's following your stories on SnapChat or Instagram. The superficiality of these constant but distant encounters are as satisfying as that low-calorie granola bar when you would rather have had a full meal.

One thing I learned in becoming involved in traditional West-African drumming is that it presents an opportunity for connection on many levels. You are engaged in a physically demanding endeavor with others. It requires one to be fully present, actively listening to others play their parts, and the responsibility and dependability of you playing your part. It generates joy, and sometimes frustration. In a well-led group, community emerges on a mind-body-spirit level through all this intense engagement. When you are in a relationship that engages mind, body, and spirit, that is pretty amazing! I don't believe you get this from Twitter, and I would also argue you get far less of it from drum circles, as discussed above.

Let me also say that drumming is not a panacea and will not be a good fit for everyone. I still encourage a healthy trial of this activity before saying it's not a good fit for a particular client, as resistance can be loud and persistent and it can be all too easy to give up without giving it a chance. For reasons such as those discussed above, music is not healing nor pleasing for all people, but it certainly is for many people. There is no one-size-fits-all approach.

Plan for the book

Readers will want to acquaint themselves with the lingo of traditional West-African drumming and other forms of drumming discussed in these pages. For this purpose, there is a glossary at the back that includes key terms, so you might want to peruse that first if you are unfamiliar with traditional West-African drumming and other drumming conventions.

The book starts by providing cultural context as I interview respected and accomplished individuals from three different traditions that employ drumming as a key element of collective community/ritual practice: Japanese, Native American, and West African. Building on my conversations with these leaders, I talk in greater depth about the role of culture and community as a salve for the modern malady of disconnection.

Some music and dance in Africa is specifically used for mystical healing rituals of physical and psychological ills, such as that discussed by Yaya Diallo in *The Healing Drum* (1989). Diallo says, " The qualified musician penetrates into invisible realms" (p. 145); that is, a mystical realm of the spirits. Diallo's home in Mali, West Africa, is one example of this type of healing, which is beyond the scope of this book.

The past decade has seen a burgeoning of research on the benefits of drumming for stress reduction and other biopsychosocial ills. I report on some of those findings and their relevance to the use of drumming in populations experiencing mental illness, addiction, and cultural as well as interpersonal disconnection. Spiritual dimensions of drumming as beneficial to those in need of existential grounding are also discussed.

Case studies of my work with individuals with mental illness, addiction to substances, trauma, and with at-risk youth are included in separate chapters. These serve to illustrate the principles and practices of using traditional West-African drumming therapeutically, and give voice to the participants as they talk about their experience of drumming. It is worth noting here that all the populations profiled engaged in group drumming. While it is possible to do individual work allowing a client to express him/herself on the drum where words fail, it is somewhat antithetical to the purpose of forming community, so those client interactions are not included here.

To protect the confidentiality of all my clients, present and former, I have used pseudonyms, have changed identifying information, and crafted composite characters to represent the issues and challenges I witnessed, and the successes we shared. To that end, if there is a resemblance to persons living or deceased, it is merely incidental and should not be ascribed to any individual.

I have mentioned drum vendors, websites, and drum teachers by name; this should not be read as an implied endorsement as I cannot guarantee quality of these companies, websites, nor individuals. Being an informed consumer is your best bet for getting what you need and maybe even more than you dreamed.

CHAPTER 2

Interviews: Grandfathers, Masters, Elders of Drumming Cultures

> "I am the drum, you are the drum, and we are the drum. Because the whole world revolves in rhythm, and rhythm is the soul of life, for everything that we do in life is in rhythm." ~ Babatunde Olatunji

There is so much we can learn from our drum masters, shamans, grandfathers. The drum master is not just a teacher, s/he is often a leader, a *sensei*, a spiritual role model. I have had the good fortune to study with a variety of such masters over the past 15 years, and I wanted their wisdom to be part of this exploration. Although many such elders, such as Babatunde Olatunji, are now deceased, I include them as definitive leaders in bringing traditional African drumming to the United States. Most is known, or published, about Oatunji.

Olatunji was born in 1927 in a small fishing village in Nigeria. He is credited as the first to bring African drumming to the US (although there were others before him, less recognized). He attended Morehouse College in Atlanta on a Rotary International scholarship. When interviewed, he recalled how little Americans knew about Africa; they were filled with misconceptions about lions roaming the streets, of life being like Tarzan movies. He enlightened fellow students by sharing information and teaching music and organized his first performance of African music and dance in 1953; he graduated from Morehouse in 1954. He continued teaching and performing African music throughout the US, including the publication of books and albums, until his death in 2003 (Williams, 2001).

Drumming in context: history and culture

While attending a Wula Drum retreat in upstate New York, I had the opportunity to view a very old black-and-white movie recording of the first time Europeans saw a performance by *Les Ballet Africains*.

Westerners tend to trivialize ritual and sacred acts as superstition or as an "exotic treat" for passive audiences (Wilson, 1992, p. xiii). The performers from Guinea in West Africa included drummers and dancers, and the musicians were as nimble on the stage as acrobats, leaping and spinning as they played their djembes. As the camera panned to the audience in a typical European theatre, patrons' faces showed shock and even terror as the attendees in evening attire appeared frozen in their seats. What a difference from traditional European classical music! One can imagine how these tight-laced Europeans saw the performers as "savages." According to Iyer (1998) there is a sharp contrast between the European model of concert music (everyone sits and listens; use of the body is suspect) versus the African model of playing and dancing (where the music and body movement are inseparable) (p. 42). The performance of traditional West African drumming and dance is distinct from European classical music, and classical dance forms, which, Iyer claims, are much more tightly scripted and hierarchical. Mickey Hart, drummer and author, states, "The first time the Western ear listens to African music the result is often disorientation" (1990 p. 197). Westerners expect linear rhythms; African music is polyphonic and dynamic. This shared sense of disorientation may be an equalizing factor in teaching drumming to clients, as will be explored further.

Aesthetics answers the questions, 'What is beauty?' and 'What is art?' Our sense of aesthetics is largely bound by our cultural frame. Music reflects the social, philosophical, and aesthetic values of its environment (Harrison, 1985). Thus, in teaching African drumming, one must introduce participants to the aesthetic of the region from whence the music originates, to set aside the current cultural frame and its associated values and tastes, to enculturate the students in such a way that the music is not "other"/foreign but a rich resource to appreciate and imitate. As Nketia suggests, "Drumming as a cultural activity has a meaning beyond structure…" (2005, p. 27); ie, analysis of only the music leaves one without the full picture.

We can learn a great deal and view the cultural "frame" within which drumming occurs through the field of ethnomusicology. This field allows us to understand the role that music plays in a particular culture, and the function of the musicians and other participants.

Major components of study in ethnomusicology relevant to African drumming include the following:

1. participants: musicians, dancers, others

2. relevant actions: dance movements and other actions occurring simultaneously with the music

3. relevant objects such as musical instruments, sound-producing items such as dancers' adornments etc.

4. the music, including song texts

5. body of culturally defined usages that govern musical events; occasions of performance and values defining when they take place

6. relationship of musical events with other aspects of culture

7. factors that affect the course of musical practice, such as culture contact or social change (Nketia 2005, p. 30-31)

Through such studies, we know that African music is "an integral part of social and cultural life, as well as a functional element of traditional institutions" in much of Africa (Nketia 2005 p. 242), while varying widely from one country to another, or within regions of Africa. Ethnomusicology also shows us that there are other aspects of meaning in African music: interrelations of structure and function, structure and context, structure and movement or dancing (Nketia 2005 p. 33).

The music may change in relation to contact with outside influences, but generally music in the oral tradition is slow to change. Likewise, the choice of musical instruments might also change, sometimes due to political factors (like being forced to move from one's home area due to encroachment by other ethnic groups) or simply access to materials to construct the instruments, or due to innovation. In both cases, evolution typically takes the form of incorporating the new into the old; retaining the focus of the primary historical music or instrument, and adding innovation in features or sounds. This improvisation, sometimes born of necessity, has been one of Africa's gifts.

Drumming today: Embracing world cultures via drumming

> "The Great Spirit loved the drum so much, He gave everyone a heartbeat."
> *~Navajo Elder*

In this section, I present summaries and observations derived from my interviews with drum masters/elders/grandfathers of three distinct cultural traditions: Japanese, Native American, and West African. I invite the reader to observe commonalities emerging in these interviews about what is important and valuable about these drumming traditions. The summaries are presented as follows: first, Japanese Taiko drumming; second, Native American drumming; and third, West-African drumming.

Interview: "Fushu Daiko" Taiko drumming group

Location: Morikami Museum and Japanese Gardens, Delray Beach FL

Event: "Sushi and Stroll"

Date: July 14, 2017

My primary question in preparing for this interview was this: What is taiko drumming?

Taiko is a mix of music, martial arts, and dance, presented with speed and power. According to Wadaiko Tokara:

> Between seven and ten thousand years ago, in the Jomon Period, simple taiko beats would be used to signal that the village hunters were setting out to gather food, or to signal that a storm was coming and everyone should find shelter. The taiko drums were used as a way of calling out to the whole village at one time to relay certain messages or to call a village meeting. This was used as a simplistic variation of village and town loudspeaker announcements that take place in many parts of modern Japan. The taiko were also used as a

means to pray for rain and for a successful harvest, as well as to strike fear into an enemy before battle. Since that time, taiko has been a deeply rooted aspect of Japanese history and culture. The rumbling power of the taiko has also long been associated with the gods, and has been appropriated by the philosophical beliefs and Shinto religion of Japan.

I arrived at the Morikami Museum, where I had arranged to meet Ben Miller, artistic director of Fushu Daiko, South Florida's traditional taiko drumming group. Parking lot: full. Entrance: one hundred people waiting in line at the ticket booth, sweating in the hot Florida sun (July!) to purchase a ticket for the show. The mood: electric.

I made my way backstage at the Morikami's small theatre to meet Ben Miller. The dressing rooms were filled with Fushu Daiko performers. The blue lights over the stage gave an ethereal glow to the small number of instruments in place. I found Ben in the men's dressing room and we began talking about the history and cultural context of taiko drumming. Suddenly, a flurry of activity as the rest of the equipment arrived and all hands were involved in hauling instruments into the theatre and onto the stage. Some of these instruments are bulky, weighing roughly 75 pounds. Each instrument is handled with great care, not just because of their replacement cost, but because they are revered.

As Ben headed for the stage door to bring in instruments, he told me to "grab other drummers" as he humbly demurred that "it's a team" and he clearly did not want star status. Other performers were happy to take a few moments to share their thoughts with me about taiko drumming and its role in their lives and on the larger stage of life.

I spoke with Ben, the artistic director and drummer; Yukako Beatty, a flautist and drummer who was born and raised in Japan; and Jeff Hollen, a drummer with the group since 1998. To say all were enthusiastic about their craft would be an understatement indeed. The troupe includes 14 performers, most of whom have been playing with Fushu Daiko for ten years or more.

My first question was about the role of taiko drumming in Japanese culture, both historically and in the present, and any differences that had occurred over time. Ben indicated that drumming is symbolic, memorializing ancestors through an event called the *Bon Festival*, a time to honor deceased ancestors and their sacrifices. The drumming creates a dialog within the team of musicians and between the musicians and the audience. The patterns of drumming create tensions for the audience and then release those tensions, replicating life patterns. Jeff agreed; this tradition represents the struggle of the people.

Taiko drumming has a greater degree of theatricality than some other forms, miming drama through drumming. Yukako saw taiko drumming as a form of entertainment, but reflected that Buddhist monks use drums at Shinto shrines as part of ritual and sacred practice. Jeff noted the vibratory power of the drums, with musicians forming drum patterns as a hopeful and positive form of prayer. The tradition is strong in the culture and here in the US as it has been growing in popularity since first introduced in the 1950s.

According to the Japan National Tourism Organization, drumming, playing flute, and dancing were methods the ancient Japanese used to call the soul back to the body as part of the Shinto belief system. Otherwise, when the soul leaves the body, one dies. The drummers agreed that taiko has evolved over time; it is not a static type of music.

I also asked what each drummer gets out of this activity. For Yukako, the practice is an opportunity to reconnect with her culture; it is also a stress reliever. This latter outcome was echoed by the other musicians. Ben emphasized the formation of community. The "tribal thing" the drummers create in interaction with each other is essential, creating meaningful bonds between members. The dynamic interaction between members, and the members with the audience, reconstitutes community anew with each practice and performance.

I asked what qualities are necessary to become an excellent taiko drummer. Yukako said that you must be strong-minded, and humble, because it's a team effort. Both Ben and Jeff emphasized that one must be heart-centered; playing with heart is a key characteristic. This form of drumming is a giving act; thus the drummer must be generous and exhibit *genki spirit*. You must "play with alacrity" according to Ben. You must be authentic and honest because "you can't hide it" when you are giving of yourself through performance. Jeff also echoed Ben in noting their reverence for the instruments: the drums are made of wood, cowhide, and metal; thus they give respect to the trees, the animals, and the earth that offers its resources so that drums can be created. The process of drumming includes honoring these elements.

I wanted to know how taiko drumming relates, if at all, to the concept of community. Yukako was clear that it is a representation of Japanese culture, which is collectivistic. Jeff indicated that taiko drumming was born of community; it is "the instrument of the people". The community gives thanks during harvest time with festival drumming. Taiko has also been called "the voice of Buddha" as it has been performed at Shinto shrines. The spiritual dimensions are part of this sense of community, and *animism*, which is also found in traditional West-African cultures. Ben added that their sensei encouraged the group to focus on the joy that they bring to their audiences; this joyful interaction reinforces a sense of community. While Ben's first taiko teacher emphasized discipline and technical excellence in drumming, his second teacher focused on the production and sharing of joy.

Finally, I asked the taiko drummers if they found any healing properties to their participation in this art form. Many cited stress relief, and a sense of catharsis for working through personal issues and negative emotions. Yukako's love for her instrument, the flute, transported her and she could "play for hours and hours". Jeff also mentioned the healing that comes from a process where "you give everything, become an empty vessel", a conduit of sorts for the shared energy of the group and what emerges through interaction with the audience.

Wadaiko, the circle, was about to become complete: our time was short and the troupe started assembling on the stage. I went to the auditorium to claim my seat. The auditorium was packed, a sold-out crowd as the Morikami Museum's website had predicted. We viewed the instruments on stage: taiko drums from small to enormous and a large brass gong. The anticipation of young and old was palpable in the auditorium.

Fushu Daiko grabbed our attention from the first shout: "*Kiai*!" Everything about the performance echoed what the drummers had told me: it was high energy, projecting the joyfulness of their experience in playing for the crowd. They opened with a song they called "Taiko Immigrants," followed by "Nankei" showcasing Yukako's flute skills, and finishing with "The Footprints of Chaos". The performers demonstrated their versatility and athleticism, switching between various instruments and making bold movements with arms and a wide stance of legs. They played hard, and played with finesse and subtlety, alternating moments of intensity with joyful faces. The musicians' obvious respect for each other, and the audience, was conveyed in their dignified manner with generous doses of humanity thrown in. The crowd loved it. With big smiles the troupe took their bows, and left the stage to cheers and applause. Afterwards they mingled with the crowd and talked about their craft.

The circle is complete. *Wadaiko*.

***

Interview: Grandfather Rick McBride and Cindy Mong

Date: July 21, 2017

Location: Hollywood FL, Grandfather Rick's home

I had the honor and privilege of visiting Grandfather Rick McBride in his Hollywood (FL) home to discuss the role and meaning of Native American drumming in his culture. His home is filled with Native artifacts, including several kinds and sizes of drums, mostly hand-crafted by Grandfather Rick: hand drums, round drums played with a mallet; the lodge drum; the Powwow or "community drum " that is typically played by multiple people at once while it sits on the ground; and hand-held rattles. Our conversation included commentary by his Quaker parrot, Speedy, whose opinion was voiced regularly as he flitted about. Also interviewed was Cindy Mong, a fellow participant in many of Grandfather's workshops.

What is the role of drumming in Native American tradition? According to the Akta Lakota Museum and Cultural Center,

> The drum is not just a musical instrument. To the Lakota, Dakota and Nakota people, it holds great cultural and symbolic power. They believe the drum has a life of its own, as well as its own powerful spirit. The drum is the heartbeat of the Indian Nation. It carries the heartbeat of Mother Earth and calls the spirits and nations together. Native Americans believe the drum often helps bring the physical and mental side of a person back in touch with his or her spiritual side. Just like many things in the Native American culture, the drum is used to bring balance and renewal to a person through participation in dancing, singing or listening to the heartbeat.

Native American drums played an important part in tribal ceremonies, celebrations and spiritual festivals, according to website Native Net. "These Native American drums are recognized as their own living entity and symbolize a strong tie with the creator. To many Native American tribes the Native drum contains thunder and lightning, and when it is beaten it helps to get the creator's attention and it also helps contact the spirits of the Native American forefathers."

Many tribes had a 'drum keeper', usually the oldest son of a selected family, who watched over the sacred drum. This was a significant honor. "The Native Americans look at the drum as a living and breathing entity; they believe that the spirits of the tree and animal that the drum was made from live within the drum. They also believe that the beats of the drum help call out to these spirits to protect and watch over them." (Native Net).

These drums were extremely important to the Native American tribes, and there were many sacred ritualistic rules surrounding a drum. Many Native Americans also use hand rattles, which are similar to the drums in the aspect of playing beats and honoring spirit. The drums had many other uses, including healing ceremonies, war preparation dances and even festivals to help bring a good harvest.

Grandfather Rick McBride is a mixedblood Ani'yunwi'ya (Tsalagi, or Cherokee) with over 30 years of active involvement in these ways. Grandfather Rick maintains a website called "Mixedblood" which is "dedicated to those who are descended in part from the indigenous people of North America. The focus is Native American spirituality and lifeways geared to familiarize mixedblood and other interested people with the *Red Road* [see Glossary]. As such, lectures and workshops on the Medicine Wheel, Medicine Shields, drums, spirituality and more are presented. These are offered to everybody, regardless of heritage."

I have had the opportunity to study with Grandfather Rick over the past two years in south Florida. Teachings on the Red Road, Medicine Wheel, Medicine Helpers, and in fact building my own sacred drum were all informative and, more importantly, extended my understanding of Native spirituality and tradition. I have attended numerous healing drum circles led by Grandfather Rick.

According to Grandfather Rick, there are several roles for drumming in Native culture. The drums support the songs, which have meaning and purpose; the songs originate in the spirit world and are sung in ceremony. The energy of the songs helps us psychologically and physically. We are "drumming up the spirits," enlisting their help and guidance. The songs stir us emotionally, "wake us up." Drumming brings us closer to our heart and spiritual nature.

Cindy Mong, an experienced participant in Grandfather Rick's workshops and drum circles, added that she believes there are gender differences in the role of drumming; she thinks that women focus more on the heart energy and benefit from it. Although in current times women drum, this was not typically the case historically. Roughly 60% of Native tribes were matrilineal prior to European contact in the late 1400s, meaning that Native traditions and decisions in those tribes were female-led; however, drummers were male in traditional Native culture. Importantly, Rick added that "spirit is gender-free" although European culture tries to assign gender to the creator and to spirit.

Drumming helps us to move in harmony; for example, as physically expressed in the *Sun Dance* [see Glossary]. In this process we are able to detach from "normal" (restrained) modes of expression. Drumming and song enable a focused type of healing; in a healing drum circle "everyone participates in the energy."

What do participants get out of this activity (ie, drumming and song)? Echoing what other interviewees have said about drumming, Cindy said simply, "Energy and calmness." Drumming has the potential to generate positive energy, while relieving stress and bringing about grounding. Grandfather Rick noted that participants gain a sense of renewal, peace, deeper contact and connection with each other. Healing occurs on various levels: emotional, psychological, and physical. Greater clarity and a sense of balance and well-being are frequent outcomes.

Participants experience the vibration of the drum along with earth's vibration, re-establishing a connection with earth/nature and a realization that we are not alone. Grandfather Rick cautioned that participants must be open to this; if they are highly resistant and maintain their walls, they may not even stay present (physically or emotionally) to experience the benefits. If they can be open, there is great potential for breaking down emotional walls and opening to greater well-being and connection.

I asked what qualities are required for someone to be a very good Native American drummer. Grandfather said that time, dedication to learning, spiritual maturity, humility, and respect are key qualities. Drummers must understand the role and purpose of the songs and various forms and purposes of the dancing: drumming supports the songs, so they must understand the meanings and play collaboratively with others. They must respect and follow the lead drum to be in harmony; for example, a floor drum or Powwow/Sundance drum, depending on the purpose or ceremony. Cindy added that the songs are prayers; the prayers are a form of honoring as expressed by all participants. Grandfather said that here on *Turtle Island* [see Glossary], drummers must be the "hollow bone," a conduit for offering connection to spirit and to healing. In this sense, drummers must "trust the drum" as it, too, is an expression of spirit.

How does Native American drumming relate to the concept of community? "It's the glue," Grandfather Rick quickly responded. "The drum draws it all together." Cindy summarized, "Drumming *is* community."

I asked, "Are there healing aspects to this form of drumming?" Grandfather Rick cautioned me to beware of focusing only on drumming; in Native tradition there is no role for "just drumming" except on social occasions. Drumming is strongly associated with song, and ceremony. He further stated, "The healing energy is in the song." Participants don't need to understand the song to experience healing. Participants enter a "meditative state" through a focus that emerges due to the rhythm being played. "Healing is for the entire village."

***

Interview: Khalid Saleem

Date: September 26, 2017

Location: via FaceTime from Brockport NY

Over the past 15 years I have had the good fortune to learn from Master Drummer Khalid Abdul N'Faly Saleem, African Music Specialist and Musical Director
of Sankofa at the SUNY College at Brockport. Khalid has served on the faculties of Duke University and the American Dance Festival where he also performs. He has traveled internationally to the Caribbean, Europe, Asia, Africa, and South America as a principle music instrumentalist with the well-known Chuck Davis Dance Company, The Egwen Dancers, The Big Drum Dance Company of Granada, and Les Guidivoir. He is a featured performer in the Dance Black America concert film shown nationally on PBS and on commercial recordings of African music, and was part of a film documentary on the life of Dr. Chuck Davis.

Khalid has also produced an audio recording series on compact disc titled "Khalid Saleem's Percussion Discussion, Vols. 1-3" as a support guide for those interested in percussion, beginners to advanced.

Khalid continues teaching, performing, and instrument-making and repair while staying connected to the community (very important to him) via universities, public and private schools, museums, recreation centers, religious institutes, and many other personal venues. He is a strong believer in peace, love and mutual respect, and that the drums aid in bringing community together.

I had the pleasure of interviewing Khalid Saleem to broaden my understanding of the potentials and possibilities of African drumming as a healing art. We spoke via Facetime in September 2017.

My key question to Khalid was, what is the role of drumming in traditional African culture?

In most cases, Khalid believes, the African drum has many roles. They are used for healing, for ceremonies, for masquerade, for rites of passage, bringing people together. *Djembe* was originally 'ankeje' or 'ankeve' and means "bringing people together." Communication was a role of the drum, because in many cultures the drum is based on spoken language, so you speak through the code of the drum to people in neighboring villages.

Personal attributes appreciated in Africa are mastery (in the sense of power and command over music production), composure (discipline), and character (integrity) (Chernoff, 1979, p. 168). These translate to vitality in drumming, where meaning , taste, and the ability to work together effectively are valued.

The *griot*, or *jeli*, is a role that is typically passed down in families. "There is no self-made jeli as some people claim today," Khalid said. "It's generational." So traditionally musicians would play the language of that drum. "Some people today don't play the drum properly, in the language of that drum, which has a particular rhythmic structure. There's a saying, 'without the drum there's no dance.' It is important that you respect the person that is playing for you."

Drums are used in almost every aspect of life in Africa. Khalid shared that "A lot of time in the US the drummer is almost like in the basement. I let people know, 'it's easy to see the flower in bloom but it's not often that the root is recognized.' Some people become famous on the backs of the musicians."

I asked, what do drummers get out of participating in this activity? Khalid stated, "For me and others, it is a spiritual connection. It's what I feel from the rhythms, how the vibrations relate to my spiritual being. It's exhilarating; it takes me to another high peak. I used to go into the nursing homes and do a little program with the drum and thumb piano, and I would see the residents maybe laying in their beds, and they'd be slumped down, and once the drum comes or the music comes, it's like a breath of life that just went into them." He continued, "For me it's a connection, and depending on what level you are in the drumming, it takes you to another place. People hear the drum, they're curious, some want to try it, they get involved, they start on a beginning level. As they continue, they get to another level .. and when you get to that peak level, I think you experience a whole 'nother spiritual thing. It's like you see the light, so to speak. I think it brings you, as a person, together. The true trinity is within yourself: mind, body, and spirit."

Speaking of the mind-body-spirit connection in drumming, Khalid mused, "The mind sometimes has its way, the body wants to do this, and the spirit tries to tell both of them what's right. Once you start drumming, you forget about things that weigh you down, certain problems, things that pull you in a wrong direction. As you get more into it, that mind-body-spirit starts to pull you in and take you to another place."

Regarding both spirituality and respect for instruments, Khalid believes "You're dealing with different elements, like the wood from the tree for the drum. That's not dead wood. The drum maker will pray and ask the spirit of that tree to keep the life in that wood to give more life for the drum. The skin [for the drum head] that comes off the animal, there's still life in it. You're dealing with the spirit of the tree, the skin, and yourself, and the ancestors that also speak through the drum."

Revealing the purpose behind the discipline of traditional West-African drumming, Khalid explained, "Over time, there are rhythms that Masters developed that give you certain reactions, especially when dealing with a healing process. And there are chants and songs. There is music to relax you, to excite you, to get you to dance. Other instruments do the same thing. In any case, there's that spiritual connection. It opens up channels in your body and it releases certain things, unblocks passages that are blocked inside, like chakras or meridians."

For Khalid and others, the purpose is simple: "So to me, just the joy of it. It just makes you happy." The pursuit of the discipline of drumming can be challenging: "Lately I see drummers [who are trying to learn a new part], I try to get them to relax because that tension is an obstacle to learning and playing well. When I'm teaching a workshop and I see that frustration building in them, I tell them it's a process, it's not like instant oatmeal or popcorn. People are trying to get it, if they relax it will come to them."

I was interested in learning what qualities or characteristics are required of a very good African drummer. Khalid immediately responded, "The main thing is respect. Respect for the culture, for your teachers, and to show that respect. The drumming world is so wide open in many ways, and people are seeing they can make a living by teaching drumming so they take anyone, even if they don't give proper respect. Respect the instrument and the culture that it comes from." He continued, "Be willing to go through the process. Not to come with evil intent. Developing a technique to be able to make the drum speak the way the drum needs to speak. Just like playing a violin, you develop your technique, how to use the bow, the proper rhythmic spacing in the music."

Commenting on how new people can successfully come to drumming, Khalid suggested that "Having a positive attitude is important. Your attitude determines your altitude. If you come in angry you will be playing angrily and that will permeate the music and negatively affect others."

Fundamentally, Khalid says, "Respect for people is essential. Chuck Davis said 'Peace love and respect for everybody.' Be willing to share, don't become territorial. Try to learn some of the language if you're not part of that particular culture. Try to learn as much as you can. Respect for the process, and that includes understanding your part. Beginners tend to get focused on learning and playing their part; it is important to listen and to understand how your part integrates with other parts being played. Find a good teacher." [Khalid's teacher, whom he honors, was Papa Ladji Camara.]

Most importantly, I asked Khalid, how does African drumming relate to the concept of community?
"For me, the drum *is* community. It creates community. The drum is your heartbeat, it's like your heartbeat. We are already rhythmic people based on our body's rhythms, when we're here to drum, we relate to that underlying inner rhythm. When I'm playing in a park, people hear the sound, it calls them, and they come to hear it or to play. It creates community, it brings people together. The sound attracts, the rhythm attracts."

Khalid reiterated, "For me, the drums bring joy and happiness, it excites people, makes them want to dance, brings people together. At times like that you don't see color, you're just joining together, you vibe together, and afterwards they communicate together and create some kind of bond. It encourages people from disparate groups to leave prejudices behind and to start opening up to each other." He added, "Sometimes people hang back, they don't know how to get involved, but if you respect their process they come back and eventually open up. Some people have heard stories that scare them about the drums, that they are evil, are demons. But over time, it is joyful to see them open up, they listen and come closer and sometimes will get involved more directly."

My key question to Khalid about African drumming was this: are there healing aspects to this form of drumming?

Khalid emphatically replied, "Yes. Depending on the community, rhythmic vibration brings healing within, it opens up those channels. I haven't taken any medicine, not even an aspirin, in over ten years. I'm never really sick. It allows your body to do what it's supposed to do. It opens up the meridians, gets rid of blockages. In some particular cultures there are types of ceremonies based on ancient traditions with an intention of healing, there are certain rhythms that deal with that." [For example, Yoruba culture and Santeria.]

Khalid also corrected my assumption that Olatunji was the sole key figure in the origin and growth of African drumming here in the US. He encouraged me to look further into how African drumming evolved in the US. He said, "Papa Laji Camara was my teacher. He played djembe on Olatunji's *More Drums of Passion* album. He helped in spreading that. But there were also drummers playing with him that were already in the US. And Olatunji was a college student at that time, and saw the interest generated by Camara and decided to promote African drumming in the US, and then it took off." Khalid made a point to identify other key figures that brought African drumming to initial prominence in the US: "Chief Bey and the drummers that played with him back then, Charles Moore, Pearl Primus (a dancer). It came from dance companies as well."

Khalid is widely respected as a master drummer throughout the communities that he has served around the United States and beyond. Chernoff states that the role of the master drummer is not inventing new rhythms, but "giving order and coherence to those already there," (Chernoff, 1979, p. 155), and Khalid more than meets this standard. He gives order and coherence not only to the traditional West-African rhythms, but in the sense of community he engenders in his drummers.

***

What kind of repeating themes did you notice in reading about these three perspectives? Here we have three widely differing cultures and percussion representations from three continents, but there are profound commonalities: respect, sharing, community, focus on others, spirituality, communication, honoring our ancestors, collectivism, humility, meaningful interpersonal interaction, connection, healing, reverence for nature, well-being of mind-body-spirit.

All three forms of drumming derive from rich historical traditions and cultural contexts in which drumming is an honored and highly interactive practice. Each of the three drumming traditions reflects a mind-body-spirit trinity that pervades the practice of drum and dance, and promotes connection and healing.

CHAPTER 3

Culture and Community; Tribe and Tribalism

> "Where I come from we say rhythm is the soul of life
> because the whole universe revolves around rhythm, and
> when we get out of rhythm, that's when we get into trouble."
> ~ Baba Olatunji (Hart, 1990, p. 214).

Much has been written about the negative attributes of tribalism; but might there be value in finding our tribe? How are culture and tribe related? What does this have to do with community, and further, of mental health and general well-being?

The problem of disconnection

What is a "community"? Is it to be found in your city or town? In your school or your church? In the diner or pub that you frequent? M. Scott Peck, in *The Different Drum* (1987) speaks of how rare the feeling of "community" has become in the very individualistic culture of the United States. In *Bowling Alone* (2000), Robert Putnam chronicles the almost-eery devolution of US culture into one of disconnection. This didn't occur overnight, nor strictly due to social media, although that is a current factor. Subtitled "The collapse and revival of American community," Putnam identifies a stretching of the social fabric that causes individuals, and families, to become less involved in their communities. For example, he traces a continuous decrease in membership in long-standing civic organizations such as the Elk's Club, the League of Women Voters, and the PTA (Parent-Teacher Association) (Putnam, 2000, p 57). Perhaps more alarming is the decrease in participation in locally-based social activities such as playing cards with friends (p. 105) or just talking together on the porch with neighbors. At the same time, an increase in solo activities arose, such as playing video games on individual devices and watching television. Participation in organized religion has seen a similar slow decline over the past several decades. The causes of this decline in connection to our friends and our communities is complex; certainly an increase in work-hour commitments and a decrease in leisure time are part of the picture. Since Putnam's book was published, we have seen a steady increase in social media distractions, which paradoxically seduce the individual into faux "connection" via Twitter, Instagram, Snapchat, and others; however, this has served to increase the sense of isolation rather than to conquer it.

A change in how we spend our time, a shift from community-based activities to solo activities, is not the key issue here, although those organizations are indeed fighting for their survival. More important, especially for professionals interested in the mental health of citizens, is how those citizens feel about this shift. Numerous authors have written about the increasing isolation of Americans, from childhood through older adulthood. This isolation causes distress for most people, and has negative mental and physical health outcomes. Depression, anxiety, substance abuse, suicidal thoughts and actions, are all possible outcomes of this desperate sense of disconnection, combined with a sense of powerlessness to change it. Researchers Holt-Lunstad, Smith, and Layton (2010) conducted a meta-analysis of 148 studies regarding the link between socializing and both mental and physical well-being. They found that in terms of the ultimate physical outcome, a lack of social relationships and feeling socially integrated shortens the life span on a par with smoking for 15 years or being morbidly obese. In short, social isolation can and will kill you, and you have a high likelihood of being quite miserable about it in the meanwhile. Conversely, involvement in an authentic community can generate deep feelings of joy (Peck, 1987).

In 2017 I posted an article on LinkedIn called "Don't Judge Me: Group Therapy and the Myth of Non-Judgmentalness." Fear of judgment is an important sub-part of our struggle with the reality of community.

As a psychotherapist in residential treatment settings, I have often seen new clients entering the group milieu who are reluctant to disclose personal history. While disclosure in individual session to a therapist may be painful, sharing with a group of peers carries a higher degree of potential for negative judgment and anticipated rejection, humiliation, or embarrassment. A client may preface some disclosure with, "Don't judge me," and peers, especially those familiar with therapy and the mantra of unconditional positive regard, will quickly assure that individual "No, no, we won't judge you," or "There's no judgment here." I say to them, "Yes, you will be judged." And then I explain.

Starting with what we know about what some refer to as the "primitive brain," our species is hard-wired for survival. The amygdala constantly surveys the environment for threats to that survival. The fight/flight/freeze response is triggered by perceived physical threats, but also by emotional threats. While most of us aren't regularly attacked by wild tigers, we may feel that way when a family member yells or a friend says something disrespectful. In either case, the body prepares for action with the release of the stress hormones cortisol and adrenaline.

The brain doesn't distinguish between fantasy or reality, thus we may find our amygdala activated when we're in a heated conversation *that isn't actually happening*. How many of us find ourselves in an extension of a conflict with a coworker as we're driving home and imagining, "well when he says X then I'll say Y, and if he comes back at me, then I'll…" To the primitive brain, that conflict is real and we become heated. Part of what we do as therapists is to help clients, and ourselves, rein in that dramatized "spin" and remember: it's just thoughts, not reality. But the point here is that the client entering the group session with a circle of unknown others represents, to our primitive brains, a potential threat on both sides. The outsider fears the cohesive front of the in-group; the in-group warily assesses the newcomer. So why would we want to bare our vulnerabilities to these metaphorical tigers?

Tajfel's 1971 experiment using Klee and Kandinsky paintings, and Sherif's "Robbers Cave" experiment (1961) are excellent examples of the psychological tendency to identify our "in-group" and "out-groups." Briefly summarized, these researchers used either art work or an artificial point-getting game with young people who didn't know each other, and identified how they reacted with an imagined out-group or in-group. Whether in an individual or group situation, our primitive brain seeks to protect and promote the perceived in-group, and identify potential threats to our perceived in-group in order to prepare a defense, or to mount an offense. In his book *The Righteous Mind* (cited in Stephenson, 2017), social psychologist

Jonathan Haidt describes the innate craving that people have to belong to a greater whole: to "transcend self-interest and lose ourselves (temporarily and ecstatically) in something larger than ourselves." Haidt calls the ability to do this the "hive switch," which makes groups more cohesive and more successful in relation to others.

Our survival needs historically depended on the fact of strength in numbers. When a lone female chimpanzee in the wild needs the support of a group, for food and protection, she will approach very carefully from the side. She may be accepted and included in the group, or she may not only be excluded but may be attacked by group members. We are not so different from the chimps. The members of our human groups make very quick judgments because, after all, if a wild tiger were attacking, we wouldn't form a committee and deliberate about whether or not the tiger was friend or foe. Thus we have judgment shortcuts, commonly known as *stereotypes*. For our primitive ancestors (who, after all, survived long enough to propagate) and the chimps, these rapid decisions based on somewhat superficial facts were essential to our ability to eat dinner that night instead of *being* dinner. We have evolved due, in part, to our skill at making rapid judgments, even if sometimes we excluded someone or something erroneously. For survival purposes, it was better to err on the side of exclusion.

When in-group individuals react to a newcomer in a hostile manner, it's not because the in-group is composed of awful people. They're just people. We are all hard-wired to *react*. The recipe seems to be: assess, react, think (maybe) later. Thus, it is entirely normal to judge others. In this sense we are *evaluating* in a very rapid way. When we evaluate rapidly, it is typically based on superficial factors. Hmm, I see big teeth, big claws, a flash of striped fur coming this way very fast … *run!*

Many of us have been coached that when going to a job interview, you must make a positive impression in the first few seconds; if not, it's over. So we dress well, smile, give a firm handshake, and so on. What's also true is that first impressions may be inaccurate, and a mature interviewer will consider information that enters the brain *after* the first minute. When an individual in a non-death-threatening situation is unable to entertain additional data, and relies on the first-impression-derived stereotype, they may be hampered by trauma-related anxiety that doesn't allow their limbic system to "stand down", or they may have other disorders causing hyper-vigilance. Otherwise, the individual who consistently relies on stereotypes can fairly be called "judgmental"; ie, that they apply their shorthand assessment without benefit of investigating additional facts.

When we use what we have learned and apply it to our current situation, we are indeed using "judgment" but aren't necessarily being judgmental. This is an important distinction to point out to clients. Judgment can be followed by openness to further data, and in fact clients can be encouraged to proactively seek new information by asking questions, inviting newcomers to share more about what brought them to treatment, and voicing ways in which established members and new members may share certain challenges. Acknowledging the reality of judgment and its sources, ironically, can build trust in the group as opposed to the automatic denial of "no, we don't judge anyone here." As clients are accepted, even with incomplete judgments, and members own their judgmentalness, emerging patterns of distorted or self-defeating judgments can be pointed out to clients as part of their growth and development.

So in my work with clients, I acknowledge, "Yes, we are going to judge you. " In fact, part of the therapist's job is to evaluate everyone in the room. We get paid to do that. Our evaluation is for safety and for moving forward with treatment goals. An effective therapist "reads the room" and identifies potential problems, anticipates direction, and may chart a course to address exactly what's going on in the room *now*.

For group members to judge newcomers, and each other, is their right and part of our human nature. Using our judgment should not be pathologized, but normalized in the group setting. The limbic system is not easily reprogrammed. *But* we are also able to set aside our stereotypes, particularly when a client discloses with authenticity and honesty. Often that sincerity is exactly what allows the group to accept the newcomer, to embrace him/her, and to see how alike we all are with our frailties, our past mistakes, and our fears.

So what I emphasize in educating clients about judging, and judgmentalness, is that we can see and acknowledge others' faults, and even challenge their self-defeating behaviors, but still *accept* them as worthy human beings. This is what evolves in a well-run group where judgment is allowed and valued, but where judgmentalness is eschewed. Judgmentalness is a forgivable offense when followed by openness to new data and honest reflection, and its appearance represents a teachable moment in the evolution of a treatment group.

The key role of community

It might seem an overstatement to conclude that the antidote to isolation is a more vibrant connection in our communities. It might make sense here to define "community". Many years ago I took a course called "Community Psychology" with Richard Katz at the Harvard Graduate School of Education. He told a story about his research in Africa with the Kalahari K'ung. Knowing a great deal about the K'ung before living with them, Katz prepared by training for and running in marathons. He described sitting in the K'ung village, preparing to go on a hunt with the K'ung tribesmen, lacing up his sneakers as they looked on, barely containing their amusement. They, of course, were barefoot. In their world, sneakers were silly. Off they all ran, and despite Katz' training and preparation, he began to fall behind. The K'ung never slowed, but they would look back at him and smile and give words of encouragement. So what does this mean? He was respected and given his dignity, and he worked very hard to keep up with them despite his limitations. The process of hunting was important, but it was just as important to make sure everyone was included, that no-one was left behind. This is one aspect of community. Everyone looks out for everyone else. No-one gets left behind. We can respect each other despite our apparent flaws and limitations, and encourage each other to greater achievement.

It is unlikely that there is any non-dictionary consensus on the meaning of community, but a key aspect seems to be "a sense of belonging" (Putnam, 2000, p. 274). Where do I belong? Where am I accepted, and valued? This is likely to differ from person to person. An intimate sense of belonging might define a family, but certainly not all families. Our identity may be tied to an affinity group, such as the LGBTQ population, or Veterans, or people who come from blue-collar backgrounds (Kastberg, 2007). How we identify ourselves is tied to how we identify our communities, and the plural is not accidental.

How would you describe a person lacking community, lacking a sense of belonging? What would be the inner life of that individual? Those are the persons I have often seen in therapy, suffering from depression, anxiety, deep loneliness, and substance abuse. I won't suggest that drumming can resolve all those ills, but I will argue that it helps a great deal, and I will provide both scientific and anecdotal evidence of the benefits.

According to Billmeier and Keita (1999, p. 17), "Drumming in Africa is not a past-time, but a part of life. It is handed down from generation to generation. The two essential characteristics of African music are invitation to participate and social function. Musicians invite people to participate – as dancers and accompanists – as this underscores social relationships. There is no separation between musicians, dancers, or other participants." One must then conclude that community is the logical result of this integrative activity. No-one is left behind.

People come to treatment from a broken "tribe" – their problems have caused family, friends, and work colleagues to reject them or the part of them that acts out or fails in ways valued by those persons. In treatment we reassemble a healing tribe, not to replace clients' primary affiliations, but to create a transitional healing space that provides time and support to recover their essential selves and to become healthier in mind, body, and spirit. But how is this transitional tribe best constituted? Here I call upon our understandings of brain science and culture. I also provide some overlapping logic from perspectives of ethnography and neuroscience in harnessing human leanings toward tribalism.

The relatively new field of sociobiology provides an interdisciplinary understanding of how biological systems intersect with social processes and behavior. Social neuroscience examines theories of social behavior along with biological concepts to understand mental health (Cacioppo et al, 2007). Likewise, evolutionary biology and neurobiology provide slightly different lenses for understanding human behavior in the context of culture. We know that so-called "primitive brain" structures were wired for competition for scarce resources in a hostile environment (Miller, 2009, 2013). These structures focus on finite survival goals such as "hurry up and kill that [food item]". That sense of urgency may cause an individual to act first and think later about a wider context, such as the possibility that there really is no competition and there are adequate resources of food.

In today's treatment environment, survival doesn't require killing food or fighting off predators. However, the primitive brain still functions in that way. More sophisticated brain structures, presumably due to evolution, allow us to function as civilized human beings in the modern world using logic and reasoning. In working therapeutically and taking the focus of the primitive brain into consideration, the goal is not to extinguish competitiveness but to invite clients to adapt to the true nature of the social environment. Thus, we invite clients to see abundance when it is present and to consider cooperation and sharing when this is truly in the best interests of the individual and group.

Deborah Tannen's (1990) work focuses on gender differences in communication. She suggests that both males and females are competitive and cooperative. However, males tend to use communication to establish a hierarchy, while females tend to focus on consensus building. Males put effort into proving who is "better", while females put effort into establishing commonality and connection. Just as Jung posited in describing animus/anima; the male and female energy within each of us is not a dichotomy but two complementary halves of a human whole. The real goal is to provide healing space where the strengths of both women and men can be harnessed, and where the misdirection of those energies can be corrected. All clients can be resocialized to claim both their male and female energies and thus become whole.

In treatment, we have the opportunity to harness what E.O. Wilson called the "tribal mind" (Wilson, 1975). We can take the best aspects of tribal behaviors that appear to arise from the primitive brain, and direct them in prosocial ways. Robert Bly (1990) suggests that socialization in the modern world has caused men, in particular, to lose or misdirect their inborn "warrior energy". That energy can be consciously directed in spiritual ways, becoming shaman-like, strong and powerful. If misdirected, the energy becomes savage and destructive, which we see on the streets of many cities today and in the histories of clients presenting for treatment.

From a Darwinistic perspective on brain evolution, Rosenbaum (2014) suggests that men tend towards ritualistic behaviors, predatory killing, and territoriality. In both men and women there is also a strong tendency to tribalism, i.e., hostility toward people who do not belong to our immediate social groups (family, village, race, etc.). This is not all bad; we try to protect our social groups against intruders and dangers perceived by our "primitive brain". However, the implications for uniform application of this reactive mode are clear.

Luckily, our modern brains are armed with something called "neuroplasticity": the brain's amazing ability to learn new tricks, or more specifically, for neurons to adapt and pick up tasks previously performed by damaged neurons from other parts of the brain. Neuroscientist Richard Davidson says: "we know that the brain exhibits plasticity, our styles in fact can be changed through a concept I call neurally inspired behavioral interventions. There are actually interventions around that were developed thousands of years ago that turn out to be very good candidates for this, and they come from the meditative traditions" (Winerman, 2012). In treatment, we are able to teach such traditions as coping strategies for the modern world of stress and challenge. We are able to introduce a variety of coping mechanisms, including the identification of thinking errors, without inviting shame for those errors.

To allow the healing energy of the true warrior is best accomplished in a community of like-minded spiritual explorers. These clients seek to consciously manage their energies towards their higher purpose and in the best interests of themselves and their tribes. In such a community, there is space for acknowledgment of grief and loss. In Bly's seminal work, *Iron John* (1990), he suggests that "in ordinary life, a mentor can guide a young man through various disciplines, helping to bring him out of boyhood into manhood; and that in turn is associated not with body building, but with building an emotional body..." Bly (1990) calls for a creative, reflective space for males to heal through association with other males, to reclaim courage and in so doing, form the inner spiritual warrior. Treatment of men often includes building a repertoire of abilities to express emotions proactively instead of via reactive physicality. Bly says that in our culture there is an absence of true warriors, and most people have no concept of what an authentic warrior would look like or feel like. Many clients are more familiar with what a "victim" looks and feels like; they know at a profound level what guilt and shame feel like.

The metaphor of the tribe provides clinicians with a broader conceptual frame for enacting the formation of a healing community. The development of spiritual warriors within the tribe of women and men is both a noble cause and one which foments success on both practical and transcendent levels.

CHAPTER 4

Science: Background and Benefits

> "Group drumming is not about inspiring successful drumming – it's about inspiring successful living." ~ Christine Stevens (2003, p. 12)

The benefits of facilitated group drumming are becoming increasingly clear through complex studies on mood states, physiology, and changes at the molecular level. A few of these studies are briefly summarized below to illustrate the variety of beneficial effects of drumming. As there are apparently no studies to date of the specific effects of using traditional West-African drumming, these summaries are based on variations of drum-circle type drumming. We hope to build upon these positive outcomes.

Recreational music-making and bio-benefits

Maxfield's 1991 thesis, "Effects of Rhythmic Drumming on EEG and Subjective Experience", demonstrated the relationship between sustained drumming and changes in the level of electrical activity in the brain. With 15 minutes or more of drumming, participants entered an alpha wave state, usually found only in those with many years of meditation experience. (Beta waves characterize the normal "active" waking experience.) Alpha wave states are characterized by feelings of well-being and alertness while the body is deeply relaxed.

Long-term care facilities for the elderly and terminally ill or disabled have long struggled with staff burnout and high employee turnover rates. In a ground-breaking study by Bittman, Bruhn, Stevens, Westengard, and Umbach (2003), recreational drumming with staff at a nursing home facility created a reduction in burnout and negative mood states (anxiety, emotional exhaustion, depression, hostility, fatigue and confusion). Positive mood states (personal accomplishment, vigor) increased. The economic impact of these changes was estimated at $80,000+ annually for a single facility.

Neurologist Barry Bittman, with Berk, Felten, Westengard, Simonton, Pappas, and Ninehouser (2001), demonstrated that group drumming –what they call "Recreational Music Making"-- resulted in an increase in natural killer cell activity – a key to immune system response in battling cancer. Additional studies have replicated these results.

In an exciting study funded by the NIH , Bittman, Berk, Shannon, Sharaf, Westengard, Guegler, and Ruff (2005) found that drumming changes individual response to stress, possibly at a molecular level. A central component of the complex human biological stress response is the modulation of the neuro-endocrine-immune system with its intricate feedback loops that support homeostatic regulation. Studying identified "stress response" segments of DNA, they found that individuals have a "stress signature" –a unique physiological response to perceived threats in the environment. The response signature included stimulation and release of chemicals in the body, often with deleterious effects. When a group drumming protocol was introduced, subjects responded in more adaptive ways. The DNA segment that initiated the stress response appeared to be modified by the drumming experience to create a different response.

Bittman, Croft, Brinker, Van Laar, Vernalis, and Ellsworth (2013) found that psychosocial stress profoundly impacts long-term cardiovascular health through adverse effects on sympathetic nervous system activity, endothelial dysfunction, and atherosclerotic development. Recreational Music Making (ie, group drumming) is a unique stress amelioration strategy encompassing music-based activities that has great therapeutic potential for treating patients with stress-related cardiovascular disease.

Smith, Viljoen, and McGeachie (2014) found that djembe drumming in both young and older populations resulted in lowering stress and anxiety and increasing cardiovascular health. Positive results for blood pressure were detailed. The low- to moderate-level of cardiovascular exercise in drumming was more easily tolerated in these diverse populations than some more intense forms of exercise.

"When a group of people plays a rhythm, not only does each individual experience change, but the entire group moves as one to a new level: we encounter the phenomenon of synchronization. Synchronization is a central mechanism of our brain, a law of nature, and a basic human need. When people in a group move synchronistically for a certain amount of time, they inevitably feel closer to one another" (Billmeier and Keita 1999, p. 11). Building upon this community-building effect of drumming, a new study finds a physiological benefit: Sullivan and Blacker (2017) found that the subjective experience of physical pain decreased when individuals were drumming. Drumming synchronously with another person (rather than drumming alone) increased the effect (ie, reduction in pain). The authors suggest further exploration of the complex link between synchrony, endorphins, and social bonding. Interestingly, the authors also discussed similar findings in a study of dancing.

In a fascinating study on the effect of synchrony on heart rate and prosocial behaviors, McCraty (2017) found that training in techniques to increase group coherence and heart rhythm synchronization correlated with increased prosocial behaviors, such as kindness and cooperation among individuals, improved communication, and decreases in social discord and adversarial interactions. The study also showed a decrease in judgmental attitudes, an increase in resilience, and a decrease in animosity between participants. Importantly, an increase in self-regulation skills was also demonstrated. McCraty also observed an increase in collectivity and related positive action through increasingly harmonious and stable relationships in the group.

In conclusion, research shows that group drumming is more than an anecdotal "feel good" experience; it has demonstrated economic, social, psychological, and physiological effects.

Body/mind/music connections

Jonathan Burdette (2017) reported on the results of a study regarding the effect of music on the brain. Measures of fMRI (functional Magnetic Resonance Imaging) were taken while participants listened to either a musical selection they disliked, one they liked (a "favorite"), or a previously unknown piece. Specifically, Burdette found that listening to our favorite music, whether it be Beethoven or Eminem, had positive impacts on memory, empathy, and "social emotion consolidation". This was regardless of age of the participant.

Burdette stated his belief in the therapeutic benefit of music for persons with a variety of ailments. Implications for the neuroplasticity of the brain, for example, with stroke patients in rehabilitation, are strong. "Music is primal. It affects all of us, but in very personal, unique ways," said Burdette, a neuroradiologist at Wake Forest Baptist Medical Center. "Your interaction with music is different than mine, but it's still powerful" (Burdette, 2017, p. 1).

Iyer (1998) writes about the role of cognition in music-making; it involves reticular (arousal/retention) systems, the hippocampus (episodic memories), and the limbic system (emotions, behavior). Further, he says that cognitive structures emerge from reinforced sensorimotor coupling (Iyer, 1998 , p 33) of audible human motion, and environmental feedback/cues [action, thought, emotion]. This is likely due to the combination of the kinesthetic and aesthetic, much like dancing, with the addition of auditory production (Iyer, 1998).

From a more anecdotal perspective, Michael Drake writes about "Reasons to Drum" in his article, Therapeutic Effects of Drumming (2006). Here are the top 12 reasons to drum:

1. reduces tension, anxiety, stress
2. helps control chronic pain
3. boosts the immune system
4. Produces deeper self-awareness by inducing synchronous brain activity
5. accesses the entire brain
6. Induces natural altered states of consciousness
7. Creates a sense of connectedness with self and others
8. Helps us to experience being in resonance with the natural rhythms of life
9. Provides a secular approach to accessing a higher power
10. Releases negative feelings, blockages, and emotional trauma
11. Places one in the present moment
12. Provides a medium for individual self-realization.

Drumming has historically demonstrated benefits on a spiritual level, as recent studies have found. Specifically, Buddhists use drumming and the bell as part of mindfulness and meditation practice. "Symbolically, sound reaches out to sentient beings in all realms of existence—in the spiritual practice of Chöd (also known as Cutting through the Ego) the sound of the drum, accompanied by a small bell, is said by some to be the voice of the *dakinis*, carrying blessings and helping to propel meditation visualization" (Lewis, 2016). The drumming induces both mindfulness and even a trance-like state where the practitioner may find a deep level of peace. Drumming is used to induce trance in other cultural traditions as well, such as shamanic drumming in South America and ecstatic dance in the Middle East. These practices can produce a sense of rapturous well-being and even out-of-body spiritual experiences. "Used in place of the breath as a tool of mindfulness, the trance-like effect of drumming provides a point of focus that is difficult to ignore and can help to still even the most monkey-like of minds" (Lewis, 2016).

Barbara Ehrenreich has documented the history of collective joy in her book *Dancing in the Streets* (as cited in Stephenson, 2017). She argues that collective and ecstatic dancing is a nearly universal "biotechnology" for binding groups together. Physical movement—a powerful escalation of typical protest chanting—not only releases emotion, it also creates bonding, trust, and equality, dissolving hierarchy and increasing a sense of community. Similarly, drumming includes movement as essential and thus creates the same beautiful environment for growth and healing.

Obviously there is abundant research and robust findings regarding the positive effects of drumming for a variety of challenges. Now, how do we apply this information?

Why Groups?

If you have read from the beginning of the book to here, you've gleaned the important role of community in serving purposes of healing. If you're a psychologist, mental health counselor, clinical social worker, or other psychotherapist, you're probably also aware of the research done by Irvin Yalom regarding the "curative factors" of group therapy (Ballinger & Yalom, 1995):

1. instillation of hope
2. universality ("I'm not alone in my struggles")

3. imparting of information (for example, learning new coping strategies)
4. altruism
5. corrective recapitulation of the primary family group
6. development of socializing techniques
7. imitative behavior (facilitator models effective task approach skills, for example)
8. interpersonal learning (improved interpersonal relationships)
9. existential factors (meaning of life, life purpose)
10. catharsis (express strong feelings that arise in a responsible manner)
11. group cohesiveness (sense of belonging).

As a therapist, I have seen all of these factors come to life in a drumming group. The facilitator has the ability to provide a safe and supportive environment to work through challenges and frustration, and to model alternative ways of "being" within the group.

Perhaps the single most important healing factor for the drumming group is that last item: group cohesiveness. Our current cultural reality in the US is one of isolation and fragmentation, as previously discussed. Coming together in the spirit of joyful music-making that is culturally grounded is healing.

The existential factors also play a key role. Psychiatrist Viktor Frankl, in his seminal work, *Man's Search for Meaning* (originally published in 1946), showed how persons can find meaning even in the face of the most unimaginable suffering. Frankl describes being a prisoner in Auschwitz, a Nazi concentration camp. The depth of physical deprivation, psychological loss, and interpersonal cruelty were crushing. Frankl made a decision to think about that horrible experience in a different way. He assigned it a positive interpretation that would enable him to go on after the war and live a life of meaning and significance. He encouraged others who were suffering to look deeply within themselves to find meaning and purpose beyond the basic will to survive.

In traditional West-African drumming, meaning already exists. Each song has a positive meaning, a recognition of life roles, life transitions, and seasonal celebrations. Western culture values individualism and consumerism. Traditional West-African songs reflect a more simple lifestyle where wealth is not measured primarily in possessions, but in the richness of meaning and connection with one's community. When individuals are able to open up to those meanings, and to each other in the group, healing is more likely to occur.

Finally, it is important to know whether you will have an "open" or "closed" group. Briefly stated, an open group is one in which newcomers can join the group on any day, and people will be leaving the group on any given day, based on when they are admitted to treatment and when they complete treatment. A closed group is one in which all members begin on the same date, and the group ends with everyone on the same date. Either group might run continuously with no identified end date, or more likely with a time frame such as 30 days, 6 weeks, 15 weeks, and so forth. An open group is more challenging for teaching drumming because the facilitator must teach the basics every time a new member joins the group. A closed group is optimal because the group progresses in their skill-building together, and learns songs together, and at a relatively similar pace. In an open group more experienced members may be encouraged about their progress by contrasting their skill level with the relative inexperience of the new member.

CHAPTER 5

Introduction to therapeutic interventions

> "In safe relationships,
> you can trust that you will not be lied to
> and will be free of exploitation,
> where the other does not feel superior at
> your expense,
> does not betray your confidences,
> or intrude upon your boundaries."
> ~Jean Shinoda Bolen, *Ring of Power*

What will you bring?

You, the facilitator, will bring yourself. What comes with that package? Are you ready to be fully present? Will you lead the group with gentleness and care? Can you set aside your own individual concerns and challenges (hopefully because you are addressing them appropriately outside of group time)? Can you see the simple worthiness of every human being in the group? Can you also admit to your mistakes, make yourself vulnerable? Can you listen more than speak? Smile more than frown? Can you project an authentic positive attitude? The most important thing you can bring to group leadership, is you. You are the instrument. The most effective leadership emanates from within.

> Show up or choose to be present.
> Pay attention to what has heart and meaning.
> Tell the truth without blame or judgment.
> Be open to outcome, not attached to outcome.
> ~ Angeles Arrien, *The Four-Fold Way*

A note about equipment

Hart (1990) says that drums have two voices; one is technical, having to do with the materials and construction methods used to make the drum, its shape, how it's played, and so on. The second voice is what he calls the "spirit side" of the drum (p. 18). This "voice" has the potential to exude energies, to alter consciousness, to speak of the culture from whence it came, and why it is here to speak. For traditional group drumming, we're going to be realistic about our instruments and then work into the energetics of them.

Budgets are real. While some begin the process of communal drumming using upside-down plastic pails, or using drumsticks to play on metal chairs, I believe in the importance of using authentic instruments. You might need to raise funds, or seek grants, or make friends with the accounting office. It is fine to start small, for example, with five djembes, as a "pilot program." Once that gets going and the accolades start rolling in, it's time to ask for another five to expand your program. More than ten is too many for a therapeutic group; it becomes less therapeutic and more about crowd control.

In some environments and with some populations, it may be wise to purchase djembes made of synthetic materials to avoid the possibility of bacteria passing from one hand to another, although evidence suggests this is unlikely to occur. There are a few vendors of synthetic djembes in the US; they are fairly affordable and not difficult to find. Sellers of the synthetic models also sell an antiseptic spray for cleaning the djembes. If you're working with individuals with communicable diseases, or you're simply in a highly risk-averse organization, you'll want to consult with the powers that be on this.

It's possible to purchase African-made djembes from US-based wholesalers at a good price. Ask for bids from three or four wholesalers. Beginners don't need high-end drums, so basic djembes are fine. If you're working with children, it's a good idea to purchase the smaller-size djembes (smaller circumference of the drum head, shorter height of the drum) but don't buy toys or so-called "festival" djembes as they won't last and producing a good sound is not likely to happen. It is great if you have the resources to buy a set of dunduns, and cowbells, which are essential in true traditional West-African drumming, but they aren't essential to starting a drumming group.

The facilitator must have a good djembe that distinctly makes the sounds you're trying to bring out in others. I've often said that my first *good* drum was like Harry Potter finding the right wand – I just knew it. Hart (1990) similarly suggests, "If the translation between inner mood and drum membrane is perfect, then you know it instantly. *Ahhhh*" (p. 117). He adds, "All sense of the present moment disappears, the normal categories of time become meaningless. Your mind is turned off, your judgment wholly emotional. …You fly like a bird. When the rhythm is right" (Hart, 1990, p. 118).

The djembe is traditionally played standing up, using cloth straps that go over the shoulders and back, and the drummer straddles the djembe. Most teachers in the US teach students in a seated position. Especially for new drummers and smaller drummers, this is probably the best idea. You will want a sufficient number of *armless* chairs. Armless is the only acceptable choice, because drummers will accidentally bang their elbows on chair arms in pursuit of the finest sounds. Folding chairs are fine.

I also provide two additional things to my drummers: hand sanitizer, and hand lotion or shea butter (traditional). Drum heads don't like dirty hands, nor dry hands. If you're working with children, it's a good idea to get them in the habit of washing their hands before drumming. I have literally had to wipe jelly donut goo off a drum head more than once (same kid).

You want to set up your group space with the chairs either in a circle, or a "U" shape with the facilitator at the top of the "U". Many indigenous cultures utilize the circle as the optimal way to respect nature and honor our ancestors. Think of the "wheel" of Native Americans, with the four directions also representing air, earth, fire, water. In *Where the Bodies are Buried,* poet Janice Mirikitani writes, "… in the circles where we face ourselves, we listen like a miracle, and I reclaim the song which is mine…" (Bolen, 1999, p. 2). Setting up classroom-style in rows is antithetical to the idea of creating a community vibe. The circle implies that this is intimate, connected space where all are honored and each contribution is valued. Plus, you want each drummer to be able to hear their peers; as the group progresses, that will become more and more important. I find that for many drummers the ability to make eye contact with their peers is also helpful, to be able to see each other smile in enjoyment and encouragement.

You need a storage space for your drums. If you're in a treatment facility, chances are that the room you drum in is probably used for other therapy groups at other times of the day. People who are unaware of the value of this precious resource may treat the drums inappropriately. So, they need to be stored away someplace safe and accessible to you. Again, make friends with the maintenance staff who will know of such a place. Educate staff about the need to treat the drums with reverence and care.

Practice. New drummers need to practice. Many, if not most, will not have access to a djembe outside of your group or class. I encourage them to practice either on their thighs (tapping out the rhythms), or on a flat surface such as a table or desk. If they are hitting their hands on a solid surface, it's a good idea to pad the surface with a hand towel. The padding also helps to prevent others from getting really miffed at the noise!

One more preliminary intervention is critical to your success: plan how you're going to involve group members who may have physical limitations. For example, I have worked with older adults post-stroke who may have command of the muscles on one side of their body, but not the other. I have worked with an individual with cerebral palsy whose movements were not always within his control. Persons with arthritis may have painful joints that preclude them from striking a drum head with their hands. In these cases, having a bell that can be secured to a stand or back of a chair and struck with a striking implement in one hand may be workable. Having a stick drum (dundun, kenkeni, or sangban) that can be played with one hand may likewise serve to accommodate an individual with moderate physical limitations.

In fact, with peer support, I have witnessed some group members becoming one-handed rock stars within the group. Their peers identify this person and his/her unique role as important to the functioning of the group as producers of pleasing music. This often evolves in ways that are surprising and satisfying to all involved. This is a huge boost to the individual's confidence in his/her ability to contribute despite mobility restrictions. That individual is able to be present as a whole person; the disability or impairment is accepted as part of who they are. Of course the plan you devise will

depend on the individual and any unique impairments. I strongly
suggest you meet individually with that client to co-create the plan
for their participation *before* they are incorporated into the group;
this is not to give them an "out" but to find a way that they can
participate meaningfully and "belong" in the group with their peers,
and also to deal therapeutically with any residual feelings of shame
due to the impairment(s).

Getting organized, getting started

Now that you've got your equipment, you have to figure out where
to have your drumming group or class. Obviously you want to make
sure that the significant decibel level is not going to bother others in
your building. Some outdoor venues work well; others have noise
restrictions. Check it all out in advance.

If you work in a healing organization, you of course need to "sell"
the drumming idea to your Clinical Director or other person in
charge of allotting time in the schedule for groups. There is plenty
of data in this book to substantiate the positive effects of communal
drumming, and more being generated even as you read these words.
You will need to educate that decision-maker about what is
appropriate to creating a communal drumming group.

Group screening is important and rarely an option in a treatment
facility. In the typical treatment setting, the people who are in your
group are whomever the boss decides is going to be in your group,
often based on convenience of scheduling rather than on therapeutic
need. In those cases, of course, you do what you can. Any group-
counseling textbook, or a SAMHSA TIP sheet (Center, n.d.), will
provide an outline of the factors you should consider when you do
have the opportunity to screen and select group members and the
process for doing such screening.

For drumming in particular, there are two types of clients I would be
reluctant to have in my group without detailed knowledge of their
histories: persons with psychotic disorders, and persons with Post-
Traumatic Stress Disorder (PTSD). As Barry Bittman stated in a
HealthRhythms training many years ago, a person who is actively
psychotic may interpret the beating of the drums as "the devil
coming up the stairs from hell to get me." That might provoke a
violent outburst in that frightened individual. On the other hand, if

that person is doing well on anti-psychotic medication and has otherwise been observed to interact appropriately with others, it might be worth a try.

Similarly, the person with PTSD may be highly reactive to loud noises. Some sounds on the drum can sound like gunfire or the booming of a distant explosion. For these sound-sensitive clients, drumming might exacerbate anxiety and panic symptoms, which will be counter-productive to treatment goals. Some anxiety in approaching the new task of drumming is fine; however, we don't want to inadvertently provoke a panic reaction due to unanticipated loud noises. I would want to discuss these issues with the client's primary therapist, and potentially with the client to hear their concerns and see if they want to give it a try. In situations where the client is ambivalent about participation due to such disorders, I also try to make sure there is a viable exit plan; that is, that the client has my permission to leave the group and has a specific place to go and staff member who will supervise them and work through any emergent reaction.

It is helpful to know what, if any, medications clients are taking. Again, talking to the primary therapist of each client or reviewing their medical record is strongly encouraged. Become familiar with medication side-effects. Some medications (or cessation from medications) can cause seizures. I have seen clients almost fall out of their chairs due to having just started a new medication with sedative effects. No-one needs those kind of surprises when you're trying to create a therapeutic and positive group experience. Prepare a backup plan for medical care if needed for a client who is having a problematic reaction to medication. If you're a licensed therapist, you probably also have your CPR certification and basic first aid, but you can't abandon your group if one individual has a medical emergency. Be sure a colleague is available to assist in the event of a medical emergency.

Before beginning drumming, I usually show new clients a short video that is both brilliant and evocative. The video currently has over 13 million views; it can be found on Youtube by typing in "Everything is Rhythm." The correct name is FOLI (there is no movement without rhythm), original version by Thomas Roebers and Floris Leeuwenberg, October 2010. This was filmed in Guinea, West Africa, focusing on the people of a village called Baro. Roebers states,

> Life has a rhythm, it's constantly moving. The word for rhythm (used by the Malinke tribes) is FOLI. It is a word that encompasses so much more than drumming, dancing or sound. It's found in every part of daily life. In this film you not only hear and feel rhythm but you see it. It's an extraordinary blend of image and sound that feeds the senses and reminds us all how essential it is.

Please take ten minutes now, put down the book, and watch the video before you continue reading. This video immediately generates an appreciation for the instrument (the djembe) and for the culture from whence it comes. I ask the clients what they noticed in the video, and this generates some discussion; I bring other details from the video to their attention and quiz them on several aspects, such as what the djembe is made from, how it is made, who makes it, and this leads into some additional relevant education about the cultural context of our drumming. Creating this positive framework really contributes to a positive approach for the anxious newcomer.

I also tell newcomers my rules for participation in our drumming group:

1. You cannot leave the group unless there is a dire emergency.

2. It is okay to be skeptical as long as you bring an open mind.

3. You have to at least *try*.

4. Treat the drums with reverence; these are sacred hand-made instruments and must be handled with care.

5. Djembes are hit only with an open hand; never a fist and not with any implements (and jewelry on fingers and wrists must be removed to protect both the drumhead and the drummer from injury).

6. Mistakes are allowed. As Bernard Woma said, "Every time one of my drummers makes a mistake, we call it a 'new style.' So please don't give me too many new styles."

7. If you do make a mistake, do it with panache and flair so it looks like you did it on purpose. Or, do it twice. Then it really looks like you did it on purpose.

8. Don't stop drumming. It's not alright to pause in the middle of a song, or a practice drill; you need to keep playing because you are part of the orchestration.

9. Posture is important. Sit up straight. Your abdominal muscles provide essential support to your upper body, which is doing a lot of work (arms and hands).

10. Listen to the facilitator (or lead drummer) and follow directions.

11. Show respect for your peers, and encourage them rather than judging them. Everyone is new at some point so your support is important.

12. Everyone has to at least attempt a solo, even if it's only one note (done with style of course). This is your time to express your unique voice on the drum.

13. Smile! This is supposed to be fun. You're not actually facing the guillotine.

14. Keep breathing. New drummers have a tendency to hold their breath due to anxiety, which hampers the brain's ability to process new information.

At the end of group, I request the drummers to put away the drums in a prearranged place for safe-keeping. If an individual is physically unable to move chairs or drums, others are expected to assist and this norm rarely has to be stated aloud.

Strategically, I have also used written evaluations of the drumming group to demonstrate its effectiveness. I would have clients complete brief evaluations at the end of a drumming session, answering questions as follows:

- What was the focus of group today?

- What did I learn about myself in group today?

- How can I apply what I learned today in group to me?

Clients could respond anonymously; the idea was not to identify a particular response with a particular client, but rather to get a sense of how the drumming group was helping clients to heal and to grow. I would compile the responses over time and share them with my supervisor and others. This helped changed skeptics to supporters of the drumming program at the treatment facility.

Here are some typical questions or logistical issues I have faced within organizations:

I've scheduled your drumming group for 3 hours on Friday mornings.

That is not a good idea for beginners, as their hands will begin to sting and burn after about 20 minutes of striking the drumhead repeatedly. We don't want to inflict pain as a requirement. I typically recommend the group meets two or three times a week, for up to one hour at a time. Sometimes I have been able to meet four times a week. Less than twice a week tends to cause frustration as there is too long a time between sessions for drummers to remember the rhythms accurately. But once a week is better than not at all.

I've assigned 25 people to your drumming group; I know you only have 5 drums but everyone can take turns.

In a treatment center or with youth groups, this is disastrous. The clients are there because they need treatment and probably have a history of acting out in various ways. As the old saying goes, "idle hands are the devil's workshop" or more secularly stated, if they're not focused on the task, they will be tempted to cause trouble. Clients not actively engaged will become a distraction to those trying to be actively engaged. Also, clients first trying drumming don't want to feel they are being watched and judged by their peers. In other settings, if clients have paid to be part of the drumming group, having them sit out for a good chunk of time will result in some very dissatisfied customers.

Your group will be in the room next to Dr. X's (psychiatrist) office.

If Dr. X is a fan of loud music, great! But unlikely. You don't want to set this up for a big negative reaction from a power player in the organization. At the very least, you have to talk to Dr. X in advance and explain to him/her the healing purpose of your group, and forewarn that it might be a little loud, and that s/he can let you know if it's too loud and you will make alternate arrangements.

[Unspoken] I'm using your djembe as a side table for my cold beverage.

It's important to educate others in your organization about how and why we treat the drums with respect. Financially, it is unwise to mistreat the drums, as it costs about $150-$200 to have a djembe re-headed. The organization (presumably) has invested in this resource and we want to protect it.

We need to use your group room today for Mr. Special's Special Presentation. You can drum with your group outside.

Depending on the nature of your healing organization, you may need to intervene here to protect your clients' rights to privacy and confidentiality. While it might be lovely to drum in the park, then their affiliation with you and your organization may suddenly become public information, and that is ethically inappropriate.

Since your drumming program is so successful, we'd like you to perform at our next Board of Directors meeting (or conference).

This has happened to me twice; once it meant they wanted a solo performance from me and another time it meant they wanted the client group to perform. On the latter count, of course we will not compromise the clients' confidentiality by having them perform publicly. (It is an option to ask the clients if they wish to perform, but have them sign a statement indicating they understand that their right to privacy may be compromised.) I will not perform as a solo artist; that is antithetical to the whole idea of drumming as a community activity. I have done conference presentations with drumming, but I include other participants in the drumming, often non-client volunteers from my outside drumming life or from the audience.

I can, and will, direct a person to leave the group if they refuse to participate, are egregiously disrespectful to peers, or if their behavior is a distraction to others. This is grounded in the concept of building a community of mutual respect and engagement. If an individual isn't "in the mood" for drumming on a particular day, I offer them the option of dancing to the drumming, which is culturally consistent. Sitting slumped off to the side looking bored is not an option. I have seen quite a lot of interesting dancing this way, as some clients find it liberating to be able to move in response to the sound of the drums. Typically the person's attitude turns around when they dance and the drummers vocalize encouragement and appreciation. I don't pretend to teach African dance as I'm not at all qualified, and neither am I a dance/movement therapist, but for clients with a variety of mental disorders, providing freedom to move their bodies in dance can be both therapeutic and joyful.

Approaches to teaching drumming therapeutically

New learners need to be acquainted with the basics: how to hold the drum correctly, hand placement, how to warm up to avoid injury. The three basic djembe sounds are taught: bass, tone, and slap. We might do some simple drills to allow the learner to see how simple it is to do these, but also not so easy to create the sounds consistently and rhythmically. I typically share with the group that I am not a master drummer; I tell them what I was told many years ago: you're a beginner for your first year of drumming; then you're intermediate for the next 17 years. So I'm still intermediate. This helps them to not be so intimidated by what I can do, as I have humbled myself and placed myself in the appropriate context as someone who continues working on technique and learning songs and practicing to improve my drumming skills. As stated previously, the use of an inspirational video helps get some motivation percolating.

Historically, traditional West-African drumming was learned orally. It was not written down, as is orchestral music for woodwinds and brass. In Africa, music is learned as passed down generationally by oral tradition or by participation. An Akan proverb says, "one does not have to make a special effort to learn the tune of a song that is current" (Nketia, 2005, p. 242). The lack of need for effort in learning, in Africa, is probably due to each fetus "hearing" the songs during gestation and at every developmental stage post-partum, since the music is omnipresent in daily life.

In the present era, many teachers use a "grid" system of music notation for teaching drumming, but this is certainly not traditional. Khalid Saleem pioneered the use of mnemonic devices to teach traditional West-African drumming. His philosophy is, "If you can say it, you can play it," and he has created instructional CDs using this approach. Musical cognition is analogous to linguistic cognition in the processing of information (Iyer, 1998 p. 19); it can be compared to the use of timing in speech (language delivery) (p. 20), with notes given emphasis just as words/syllables are given emphasis. Thus, Saleem has created words and phrases that assist the learner with remembering the parts so they can practice and play them correctly. Particularly for persons unfamiliar with the polyrhythmic sounds of traditional West-African drumming, using mnemonics is very helpful.

Example 1: "I (pause) can (pause) play-this-rhythm." [Bass, bass, tone, tone, tone-tone.] This is a djembe part for the song Kuku, which was played when the women in a village returned from fishing with that night's dinner. The facilitator plays the rhythm to demonstrate, and also "sings" the words so the learner pairs the rhythm correctly with the mnemonic device. Repetition is key.

Example 2 (also Kuku): "Ku-ku-bey-la". [Bass tone-tone slap.] My colleague, Doreen Cahill, a clinical social worker, heard me teaching this particular part using the mnemonic. She is an EMDR practitioner. EMDR stands for Eye Movement Densensitization and Reprocessing, a technique used to assist clients in healing from trauma. One method of using EMDR is to "tap it in" – that is, the client says specific healing words and simultaneously taps on their body as instructed by the practitioner. Doreen shared that my use of mnemonics while drumming was another form of "tapping it in." Thus, I experimented with using a different mnemonic for "Ku-ku-bey-la". With my group of addicts in recovery, I taught them "Clean-and-so-ber". As you can see, it has the same number of syllables and the correct inflection to replicate the same djembe part, while reinforcing their recovery.

I teach everyone part 1, then teach everyone part 2, then divide the group in order to have both parts played simultaneously. First, I demonstrate with one other drummer how the two parts fit together; the disparate parts are having a "conversation" with each other and this musical dialog is essential to the orchestration. With new learners, it is very difficult to play a part while others play a different part; this tends to create chaos. Mickey Hart says that only when the drummer can listen to two rhythms at once (his own and another's) without losing his place can he be considered a true African drummer and able to play with others (1990 p. 197). Thus, training begins with one rhythm and proceeds to add from there.

With time, the drummers are able to not only play their part, but also listen to the other part and understand how the two (or three, or four) parts fit together. It is often helpful for clients to realize that from apparent chaos, order may be found. The structure of the music is comforting; it helps them contain their inner chaos while they are learning new coping skills. "The power of the music comes from the conflicts and conversations of the rhythms, from vivid contrasts and complementary movements" (Chernoff, 1979, p. 160).

In this process of playing in a group, clients learn to make *micro-adjustments*. Harvard physicist Eric Heller and postdoctoral fellow Holger Hennig studied the millisecond errors that Ghanian drummers make normally (Hennig, Fleischmann, & Geisel, 2012). Humanly-produced music (ie, not governed by a metronome nor computer software) is characterized by tiny adjustments in response to the other players' music production. If humans play rigidly, like a metronome, it is likely to be unsuccessful and listeners find it somewhat unnerving and not pleasing to hear (Hennig et al, 2012).

Deviations in human rhythmic production are fractals, following the same mathematical principles as do snowflakes. These deviations are preferred by the human ear. For persons suffering from mental disorders, instruction in microadjustments is very positive to their interpersonal interactions, because the rigid social approaches some may have been using tend to be very off-putting. In order for clients to make this connection between drumming and "life", I am explicit in pointing it out to them and inviting comparisons between being rigid in interacting with others, versus making microadjustments.

When playing multiple parts, as is the case with all traditional West-African songs, connections in the brain are strengthened. Specifically, the corpus collosum allows the left side of the brain to communicate with the right side, and vice versa. In a very entertaining talk given by Deborah Tannen, an expert in gender differences in communication, and poet Robert Bly (1992), Bly describes the corpus collosum this way: in females it is like a 6-lane expressway going at top speed. In males it is like a narrow dirt path full of rocks and potholes. In reality, it might not be quite so different based on gender, but certainly there are person-to-person differences. From the perspective of Eastern philosophy and practice, through these kind of stretches we are integrating Qi (energy) through the movement of yin and yang energies throughout the body, mind, and spirit, bringing harmony and flow.

One of the ways I try to get clients to stretch their cognitive abilities is to ask them questions while they're playing a particular part. Once they get in a groove, solidly playing the part, I tell them that I'm going to ask them some questions, and they have to *keep playing* while they answer the questions. I might ask something very simple, such as "what's your favorite color" or "when is your birthday?" I might make the question related to the client's purpose for being in treatment, such as, "How many days clean do you have now?" This sounds simple, but it can be very challenging to use different parts of the brain at the same time: producing music and doing mathematical computations. I am role modeling for them when I do this, because I'm also playing while formulating and asking questions. Clients often glow with pride when they are able to develop enough drumming skill and cognitive flexibility to be able to play and talk at the same time.

I always explain the meaning of the song we're playing. Most songs have a meaning related to life roles, life transitions, or life events. There's an occasional song that is simply celebratory; ie, let's party! The meaning of the song brings cultural context to our playing of it; it is not just pointless drumming. The drumming is situated as a primary means of keeping our "community" together. The process allows each group to begin to see themselves as members of a unique community with interdependence at its core. If you don't have access to a course in ethnomusicology, a helpful publication featuring master drummer Mamady Keita, working with Uschi Billmeier, is *A Life for the Djembe*. This book includes a CD, and provides explanations and musical notation for many songs of the Malinke people of Guinea. It includes information on history, culture, and photos of important rituals (that would be accompanied by drumming and dance). This will help you get started in understanding the importance of drumming in traditional West-African culture so you can share it with others.

At the end of each drumming session, I set aside the last five or ten minutes to ask each drummer to say what they liked most about the session, and what they would like to see changed or improved. This public voicing of "what's good" often becomes about the individual sharing how they feel about their improvement in skills, or how they are seeing the effects of the drumming on their interpersonal interactions within or outside the group. The suggested improvements are invited not gratuitously; if the group members have suggestions that I can accommodate, I generally will do so. I also let them know that my view is that the way you drum is the way you live. In other words, how a individual approaches drumming, how they participate as a member of this community, tells me a lot about what their challenges are in their life, and how they handle it. I might say to a drummer, for example, "how is your difficulty focusing on what we're doing right now, representative of your life outside of drumming?" We might be able to productively address that in group, or at least bring insight to that individual about the consistency of problematic behaviors that they take with them wherever they go.

Acknowledging obstacles to healing

Many therapists use a strengths-based approach to mental health treatment; that is, we identify the resources and qualities that a client has previously demonstrated as useful strategies, and bring these to bear on whatever might be the current challenges. We bring to the client's attention that, indeed, they have skills and proven tactics that can be applied to their unique problem. Often a client feels overwhelmed by their problem or issue and is unable to see what they might be able to do to address it. There are literally hundreds of therapeutic techniques therapists use to engage clients in a healing and growth-promoting process. Realistically, however, there are obstacles that clients also bring with them to therapy. Dr. Stan Hyman, a psychotherapist in south Florida, identifies the top ten barriers to self-growth, as follows:

1) Fear: It may sound obvious that fear would be number one on the list but many people don't experience it that way. They may rationalize their reluctance to make changes by interpreting their excuses as valid reasons. It is often only through taking an honest personal inventory or thorough self-examination that a person realizes that his fears have been driving him.

2) Denial: Others may have suggested that you need to change (maybe you're too angry or stubborn) but you are not hearing it. You prefer living in your own world of fiction despite what people close to you (and even, perhaps the little voice inside your head) have said. Personal growth will not be possible if you think it is unnecessary for you to make changes.

3) Pride: There's nothing wrong with being proud, as in being proud of your accomplishments. However when someone has an inordinate opinion of his own importance and carries a sense of superiority over others, it will prevent him from keeping an open mind about change and growth. Pride sometimes prevents people from being willing to admit they made a mistake, thereby learning from the experience.

4) Defensiveness: Being overly defensive is a signal to others of your insecurity. A person who is excessively concerned with guarding himself against real or imagined criticism is not able to grow. His defensiveness closes him down and he becomes a prisoner in his own prison.

5) Not taking responsibility: Repeatedly blaming others or circumstances for what happens in your life is a way of avoiding your own responsibility. To experience self-growth you have to be ready to take the heat. Blaming others can create the conflict you need to deflect the focus away from you and onto someone else.

6) Lack of self-discipline: If you have lofty ideas about the things you would like to achieve and the person you would like to become but lack the self-discipline to accomplish those things, you will always be disappointed in yourself. There is no reaching the top if you are not willing to make the climb.

7) Lack of motivation: It is easy to say that you would like to do something (for example: exercise, learn a language or get better at being in a relationship) but until you understand why you want to do something you will likely not accomplish it. Being truly motivated creates a powerful force or _drive_ that can propel you to achieve what you want. Many people just think they should want something and create a fantasy around the thought. Try answering this: What do you want that you really cannot live without?

8) Lack of goals: It is the old story of: "If you don't know where you are going, how are you going to get there?" To achieve growth you need to know what you want and map out a course to get it. Many people resist creating and writing down goals often because they have simply not gotten into the habit. Start small and build your goal setting skills.

9) Negative/Pessimistic attitude: This is not the same as having healthy skepticism. Having a negative/pessimistic attitude creates an internal state where few, if any, options exist. Expectations of only the worst sort of outcomes cloud

the mind and hamper the possibilities of growth. The spirit is drained of inspiration and the person is stuck. Learning to creating a healthier attitude will open up your options.

10) Lack of support: If you surround yourself with negative/pessimistic people you are unlikely to achieve personal growth. If you do not have a good support system you should try to develop one. It is hard to go it alone. To achieve good and great things in your life you need the support of good and great people (Hyman, 2017).

To these I would add sabotage, and self-sabotage. Believe it or not, family members of persons with mental disorders are often subconsciously comfortable with the status quo: the identification of the client as The Person With A Problem. When therapy starts unraveling some family secrets, for example, which makes loved ones appear less stellar than they prefer, they may sabotage the client's progress. This takes many forms, and generally I have found that sabotage is an entirely unconscious process in the minds of family members. Likewise, clients with a very low sense of self-efficacy and lacking belief that their changed behavior will result in different outcomes will often engage in self-sabotage. Similarly, this is a largely unconscious process but might appear as an addict working on recovery having a "slip" (using a small amount of a substance one time), or a person with a mood disorder "forgetting" to take prescribed medications. The therapist's role here is to bring these unconscious fears and resistance to the surface so they can be worked through as part of the healing process.

CHAPTER 6

Therapeutic interventions part I: recovery from addictions

> "It was but yesterday I thought myself a fragment quivering without rhythm in the sphere of life. Now I know that I am the sphere, and all life in rhythmic fragments moves within me." ~ Khalil Gibran, *Sand and Foam* (1926, p. 2)

For readers who are unfamiliar with substance use disorders and treatment for such disorders, a brief overview is provided here. More thorough information is abundantly available from the websites of the Substance Abuse and Mental Health Services Administration (SAMHSA), the National Institute on Drug Abuse (NIDA), National Institutes for Mental Health (NIMH), the National Association of Alcohol and Drug Abuse Counselors (NAADAC), as well as numerous articles and books on the topic.

Who comes to addiction treatment? The variety of persons coming to treatment is quite diverse, from teens to elders. In fact, SAMHSA reported in 2010 that the rate of elders (age 50 and older) coming to treatment for substance abuse more than doubled from 1992 to 2008 (Substance abuse, 2010). With the advent of mental health parity law requiring insurers to cover mental health treatment, and with that substance abuse treatment, you might see anyone there. Demographics vary not only with age, but socioeconomic status, race, religion, ethnicity, and level of education. Substance abusers may be stay-at-home moms, teachers, first responders, psychologists, nurses, doctors, lawyers, and any other profession you can name. Treatment is available to those with money, or those with health insurance. Treatment is available sometimes to indigent persons, but there are often waiting lists at free/public health centers, and group sizes are typically large so the treatment is far less personalized. There are "luxury" treatment centers that aim to make clients as comfortable as if they were on vacation in a resort, with spa treatments and other accoutrements of easy living.

A substantial proportion of people with substance abuse disorders also have mental health problems (for example: depression, anxiety, bipolar disorder, trauma). "For patients with mental disorders who are seen in specialty treatment settings, about one-fifth have had a substance abuse disorder within the past six months" (Regier et al., 1990). For these individuals, treatment is a complex process that will only be effective if both the substance abuse disorder and the mental disorder(s) are addressed simultaneously. It stands to reason that if the mental disorder is untreated, substance use will likely resume upon discharge from treatment; if the substance use is untreated, the mental disorder will likely not respond to treatment.

What are the substances of abuse affecting those who come to treatment? Again, it varies widely, and often an individual is abusing multiple substances before coming to treatment; those individuals call themselves a "garbage can" because they'll take anything to get high. Alcohol is often a substance of choice, so is heroin, crack cocaine, the list goes on.

Why do people abuse substances? The common myth is that individuals "self-medicate" and sometimes this is true, but not all the time. Some people try a particular substance out of curiosity, recreationally. I have yet to meet a person who intended to get addicted. Many factors go into the use of substances. For example, alcohol is a legal drug in our society for those ages 21 and older. It is socially acceptable. If a medical doctor prescribes an opiate medication for pain control, it is socially acceptable. Sometimes individuals are too embarrassed to tell their doctor that they have developed an addiction to the pain medication; when the doctor discontinues the prescription, they may shop for another doctor, or turn to buying the drug on the streets. When/if that becomes too expensive, as it typically does, opiate users often turn to the cheaper alternative: heroin. Yes, grandmothers and grandfathers use heroin too. The stereotype of the drug abuser is some dirty homeless person, and that is rarely accurate.

What types of treatment are available? There are both inpatient and outpatient treatment options. As a first step, many individuals will go to a detoxification ("detox") unit that provides medical supervision to prevent harm due to seizures and other medical issues caused by withdrawal from drugs such as alcohol or heroin. Inpatient treatment may be mandated by a court; it may be coerced by family members; it may be chosen by an individual who truly wants to recover from their addiction. Inpatient treatment is intensive and occurs in a facility that provides housing and meals, as well as access to medical care. The typical inpatient program is a minimum of 30 days. Outpatient treatment is typically far less intensive. An individual may attend therapeutic groups three or four times a week for two or three hours at a time as they grapple with the realities of facing work, relationships, and financial issues without their usual stress reliever: drugs. Of course, many individuals forego formal treatment and attend free support groups provided by Alcoholics Anonymous (AA), Narcotics Anonymous (NA) and others. The effectiveness of participation in any of these forms of treatment is inconsistent, given a relapse rate of somewhere between 65-95%. One study indicated that relapse was related to education level, with an overall relapse rate of 58% (Blum et al., 2014) and the best outcomes are garnered by those with higher education levels.

Common areas of deficit

I have often said that when addicts come to treatment, they all exhibit features of Antisocial Personality Disorder (APD): they are extremely self-focused, and show no authentic signs of remorse for having hurt others. While some eventually are diagnosed with APD (a very small percentage), most become less selfish and more remorseful as their brains shed the toxicity of the chemicals that have flooded their brain. In his excellent book, *Addiction and Change*, Carlo DiClemente writes that the addict's regulation of behavior appears either in poor control or "out of control" (2003, p. 46). Further, DiClemente states that the individual who has developed dependency on a substance(s) continues their use despite negative feedback or negative outcomes, and that the substance has become an essential coping strategy for that person. So, for example, a person in active addiction (ie, the person is actively seeking and using the problematic substance) might steal a precious memento from their grandparent in order to pawn it for money to buy drugs. In that moment, their primary goal is to address their own perceived needs. They show little or no empathy or compassion for the grandparent who will be highly distressed to find their irreplaceable possession missing. Later, as the toxic brain soup recedes, a good deal of shame will be experienced by the addict as they face the harmful outcomes they created. This shame often creates an urge to use, due to poor coping skills for dealing with difficult emotions, thus creating a cycle of recovery and relapse.

In addition to these typical signs of drug dependence, the addict typically has become estranged from important relationships such as family and friends, often due to their abuse of those relationships (stealing money and other possessions). They make a lot of promises to those loved ones, and then fail to keep their promises. I have seen clients who are in treatment for the 19th time at age 19, and for the 34th time at age 57. You can imagine how betrayed and burned-out loved ones can become in the face of so many failed treatments. For families, it is emotionally and financially depleting.

Addicts can find themselves very socially isolated, hanging out only with other addicts because they have burned all their bridges during their years of using drugs. One wife told me, "Yes, I'm his wife, but his real wife is heroin." A female crack addict gave up custody of her toddler because she saw the child imitating her actions of crushing pills between credit cards and sniffing the drug. Frequently the drug of choice becomes the beloved mistress; the addict will do anything and everything to keep this mistress in his/her life, and she is a harsh mistress indeed, for the addict will lose everything in pursuit of this love object.

The addict spends a good deal of their waking hours in pursuit of the love object, and this often causes employment problems; specifically, frequent absences or lateness cause one to get fired. I have had more than one client who was caught doing drugs on work premises and was fired on the spot. Being an addict is very time-intensive; the addict must get the money necessary to purchase the drug, and must find a person who has the drug and will be available to sell the drug. Then s/he finds a place to use the drug. For alcoholics, again, this is easier because purveyors of alcohol can be found very easily and it is only criminalized when the individual gets a DUI or otherwise causes direct harm to others. The heroin or meth addict often finds themselves in very risky environments to buy and use their drug of choice. I have had clients who had been beaten, stabbed, and shot; who contracted Hepatitis or HIV from using dirty needles, who had huge abscesses at injection sites now infected, or MRSA (an antibiotic-resistant staph infection) that required hospitalization. In our current era (2018) the overdose death rate has become truly shocking. Suicidality is also a risk factor in this population as hopelessness sets in.

Less has been written about the characteristics of the individual coming to treatment for substance abuse. The "top ten" stated by Dr. Hyman in a previous section start with fear, which is a significant factor with this population, as are most of the others on that list. There is a lack of self-knowledge, and by this I mean an awareness of one's own core values, personality type, and other characteristics. Along with this I often see a lack of direction or sense of purpose, and profound spiritual disconnection.

There are often significant deficits in pro-social behaviors. The addict often demonstrates anti-social behaviors and has been practicing that during active using. Such antisocial behaviors include criminal activity, such as stealing, drinking and driving, physical assaults on others, prostitution/pimping, working as a "drug mule" moving drugs from state to state or even from country to country. It is not unusual for an addict to have felony convictions prior to treatment, or charges pending. They may also face charges of domestic violence, child abuse or neglect, or elder abuse.

Some may lack appropriate assertiveness or refusal skills, such as the simple "No" when you are offered a drink or drugs. "Assertion is the behavior or trait that allows people to appropriately express their personal rights and feelings" (Lewis et al., 2002). Assertiveness can be contrasted with less successful behaviors, such as aggression, passivity, or passive-aggressive behaviors (Stevens & Smith, 2009), all of which we see in this population.

Many addicts lack appropriate boundaries. Simply stated, boundaries are "where you end and I begin." Persons with healthy boundaries tell others to back off when their personal space is entered, and say "no" when asked to do something they don't really want to do. Poor boundaries are often a result of never having learned, or been given permission to have, healthy boundaries. Boundary violations in childhood are over-represented in this population; specifically, there are far more victims of childhood sexual abuse in the addict population than you would normally find in the general population. In treatment clients often tell someone (usually a therapist) for the first time about having been molested or sexually abused as a child. Sometimes they have been sexually assaulted as an adult, but didn't report the rape because they were using drugs at the time and didn't want the police around, or didn't think they would be believed.

Addicts come with both an abundance of guilt and shame, and deficits in the ability to recognize and articulate their own emotions. Drugs or alcohol were used to become numb from overwhelming feelings. In order to reduce the urge to use, coping strategies for dealing with difficult feelings, such as shame, must be learned. Burying negative emotions is ineffective; using is ineffective on a long-term basis because the using just adds to the feelings of shame. Grief and loss are also present. Addicts have often lost everything important in their life or are at imminent risk of losing these: job, financial stability, relationship with significant other(s), a sense of belonging. Along with these, self-esteem is usually extremely low and self-loathing is present.

Paradoxically, the addict who desperately needs help and support will typically refuse to ask for the kind of help that will really lead to recovery. Humility is lacking. There is a lot of false bravado, pretending you know something that you really don't. This takes the old joke about males refusing to ask directions to an extreme level. The addict needs specific skills training in coping strategies and refusal skills, to name a few; it helps a great deal when the addict is able to say out loud, "I need help; this has gone way beyond what I can handle." Even in a group therapy session, it is a positive sign when an addict admits, "I don't know [how to repair my broken relationships, for example]".

Individual issues may include impulsivity, inconsistent behavior, and ambivalence about recovery. In other words, some addicts aren't sure they want to get clean and sober, and their impulsivity may lead them to use without thinking it through. Part of the role of treatment is to show the addict how what they're doing is making their lives worse. We tell them to "play the tape all the way through"; in other words, don't just focus on how great it feels to get high, remember all the negative consequences you experienced after the high.

Addicts are masters of manipulation. They have practiced the skill of getting others to do what they want or need, such as giving them money, helping them get out of jail, lying to others. They are the greatest salespersons on earth. I have heard many stories from parents about how they had to send the client money for the electric bill that was 3 months past due, only to find out later that money went for drugs and the electric bill is now 4 months past due. Due to all the lies, cheating, and other manipulations, the addict's credibility is very low with persons close to him/her. The people s/he needs the most are likely to keep their distance, and keep their wallets closed. When the recovering addict begins to exhibit more positive behaviors and turns to loved ones for help in recovery and are turned away due to past mistakes, their low frustration tolerance may be a trigger to use.   They are impatient and want recognition of their improved behavior before others are ready to give it. Trust must be earned.

Inertia is also an issue. Addicts become paralyzed by their recognition of how bad their life circumstances have become, how angry and disappointed their now-distant loved ones are, how their criminal behavior now limits job prospects and thus financial prospects, and how lonely and depressed they are. They have very little self-esteem and poor self-efficacy, so they get "stuck" in what AA calls "stinking thinking." This often leads to relapse, unless effective intervention occurs.

I often see a lack of balance in the life of the addict and in their thinking. Especially those who started using at a young age, have the puerile belief that life can be all pleasure and no pain. They envision a life in which all is comfort and contentment. Obviously this is non-existent. Somehow the drug "high" leads them to believe that life could be one never-ending high. In those moments of anguish they recall the high and forget all the negative outcomes they have experienced and will continue to experience in active addiction. The addict must begin to tolerate the coin of life, with one side pain and the other pleasure. There is no double-headed pleasure coin.

The old "moral" theory of how addiction develops suggests that the addict is weak, immoral, sinful. While it is true that a lack of self-discipline is often evident in a person in active addiction, we must also recognize that it takes a lot of time and effort to be an addict – as outlined above, being a salesman to get money (albeit illegitimately), pursuing the drug and dealer, evading detection, and so forth. What appears as a lack of willpower is simply evidence that the brain has been hijacked by drugs (a current, evidence-based biological theory of addiction). Acknowledging that addiction is a disease of the brain is important, and recovery is possible. We can harness the energy that has gone into drug-seeking behavior and redirect it to pro-social behavior, but it takes time and help.

How traditional West-African drumming addresses areas of deficit

As discussed above, we often find these areas of deficit in persons who are attempting recovery from substance abuse:
- Fearful
- Lack of self-knowledge, awareness of identity or values
- Lack of positive social skills
- Prideful (unable or unwilling to say "I need help" or "I don't know")
- Isolated, lonely
- Self-focused
- Lack assertiveness skills
- Poor boundaries
- Low self-esteem
- Blunted emotions
- Abundance of shame
- Impulsive
- Inconsistent
- Ambivalent about recovery
- Uncooperative or superficially cooperative
- Manipulative
- Dishonest
- Impatient
- Low tolerance for frustration
- Plagued by inertia
- Poor self-discipline
- Lack of balance, unrealistic expectations

As simple as it sounds, recognition and naming of feelings can be taught. *Radical Acceptance,* a book by psychologist and Buddhist Tara Brach, addresses this topic. Brach (2003) suggests that many of us are unfamiliar with our own feelings, especially any of the so-called "negative emotions" such as sorrow, anger, or fear. For example, if we are feeling envious of another person, we might recognize our envy subconsciously, but immediately jump over that feeling to evaluating it critically, and then feel angry with ourselves for being jealous, thus compounding the negative mind-state. Rejecting our feeling of envy is unlikely to actually remove the jealousy. Accepting it might be better; creating space to think through what is causing that jealousy might be productive.

If we're feeling frightened in a new situation but were taught to be brave and never cry, we may feel ashamed of our own fear and nervousness. Again, denying the fear will not make it go away; it just sinks below the surface of our awareness but reveals itself as continuous anxiety and emotional discomfort. Brach says we need to recognize and name our feelings inside our own head, and just accept what we're feeling, rather than judging that feeling. Feelings are just feelings. No more, no less. If we identify the feelings, they are more likely to gently subside. If we resist the feelings because of our own negative judgment of those feelings, that battle will rage endlessly. After identifying the feeling(s), we can then decide whether or not to say something out loud, such as "I felt startled when you came up behind me and yelled." That assertive statement might lead to constructive dialog and problem-solving.

In addition to the deficits that bear a direct relationship to the abuse of substances, individuals are often dually-diagnosed; that is, they have both a substance use disorder and also another disorder(s), such as depression, anxiety, or personality disorders. So there may be co-occurring deficits such as lack of focus, difficulty concentrating, low mood, extreme nervousness, and so forth. Some of these can also be improved through drumming, but most will benefit from individual therapy sessions as well.

Social skills can most easily be taught through role modeling, demonstration, and role play (Stevens & Smith, 2009). Group therapy provides plentiful opportunities for all of these, plus psychoeducation that explicitly teaches how to interact appropriately. In a drumming group with individuals who have never drummed before, fear is present in the face of a novel task. Individuals are afraid of making mistakes and being humiliated in front of others. This fear can be addressed right away.

Regaining balance in life is a process, not an event. Both in treatment and in attending AA or NA meetings, addicts hear the life stories of other addicts who are now in recovery. These authentic narratives begin to show addicts that life in recovery is imperfect; that those in recovery struggle with work, school, love, money, all the things we wish were perfect but aren't. They also see that despite the imperfection of a life of recovery, this is a far better life than what they have experienced in active addiction. In drumming, they also experience the balance between giving and receiving. First, we give our music to those dancing and listening for their greater joy; seeing the enjoyment of others gives us joy. The paradox of life, as exemplified in drumming, is that when we give generously of ourselves, we also receive.

Case histories

Case 1: Carl

Carl was a 25-year-old who had struggled with addictions for several years. His childhood was marked by an abusive father and a submissive mother. Domestic violence was a regular occurrence and no-one prevented the abuse from occurring. Carl had won the genetic lottery in terms of looks; he was tall, slender, with light eyes and caramel-colored skin and curly black hair. He had been able to manipulate many women, girlfriends and their mothers, getting them to give him money for drugs, and later, for treatment. Carl had moved from using anti-anxiety medications (unprescribed) to crack cocaine, to opiate pills, and back again. He had short periods of homelessness until he found the next girlfriend. He was charming and angry about his history. He felt cheated out of a "normal" childhood. He also felt justified in using the many women he had exploited for money and sex; they were easy marks for him and he had experienced relatively few negative consequences for his history of using drugs and cheating on women. This time, he seemed to be running out of luck and was back in treatment for the seventh time. His motivation for change was fairly low, and he also had Attention-Deficit Hyperactivity Disorder (ADHD) that would remain untreated because many of the medications prescribed for ADHD are stimulant drugs that can and will be abused by addicts. Iyer (1998) has written of the relationship of drumming to the mind's ability to concentrate and focus: "musical meter provides us with an attentive mechanism – a temporal template against which to process information in time, reducing demands on memory" (p. 18). Thus we see the power of drumming to assist in focus and attention in the individual with ADHD.

When Carl came to drumming group, he had a big chip on his shoulder; negative attitude and not motivated to try drumming. However, he stood very close to me and said, "Oh you smell so good," an obvious attempt at manipulation. His false bravado led him to pretend he was already a drummer; to save his dignity, he allowed that he was really a kit drummer and hadn't tried this kind of drumming. I encouraged him to be skeptical all he wanted, as long as he was also open-minded. Luckily, Carl was bright and capable and quickly picked up the basics. For the first week he learned the song parts for Kuku, but he would not "stay in his lane" and play his assigned part. He wanted to solo endlessly. We discussed how this might be meeting his needs for attention, but it was not the kind of positive attention he craved.

By the third week, Carl was beginning to see why it was musically important for him to play his assigned part, and only solo when he was invited to do so. The orchestration was really coming together, and Carl felt good about his role and contribution. There were many more smiles in the group as the song was sounding better each day. Carl played his part as assigned, and had his moment to shine when he was invited to solo. Importantly, he said out loud what he was learning about himself, and admitted that his initial approach to drumming (soloing whenever and wherever he wanted) was a mistake. He found that playing as a member of a community of drummers requires some personal self-discipline, and that if you do your job, you will also have the opportunity to receive positive attention from your peers.

Case 2: Jalisa

Jalisa was a very quiet Latina woman, age 35, who came to treatment for her alcohol dependence. She consistently used alcohol to numb her feelings and to "deal with life," as she put it. Jalisa had a domineering husband, and she played the role of dutiful wife. She loved her husband deeply, but her life was spiraling out of control due to her drinking. Her employment was in jeopardy, and her marriage was strained. She avoided interacting with other family members and had isolated herself from friends as she feared their judgment about her drinking. She disclosed that she had been raped as a teen and had never told anyone. Meeting her husband had been the shining light in her life to date, but she had never dealt with her sexual assault and the feelings that came with it. It took several weeks before she could uncover her anger and begin to face it without hiding emotionally. That undercurrent of anger was a huge trigger to her continued drinking and had to be addressed.

When Jalisa began drumming, she barely touched the drum, she was so hesitant and afraid of making a mistake. Her body language suggested that she was afraid I would strike her. She held her shoulders in a perpetual anxious hunch, and scrunched herself off to the side of her chair so she wouldn't be too close to the other drummers. She always sat closest to the door, as if she would jump and run at any moment. She was always cooperative, but voiced her hesitance as well as demonstrating it.

Jalisa's primary therapist was working with her on assertiveness skills, and so I collaborated with both of them to help Jalisa "attack" the notes on the drum, to experiment with being bold and musically forceful without being aggressive, which she feared. I wanted her to claim her space in the song. It was important for me to role model assertiveness in drumming and in my interpersonal interactions with all the drummers. By chance, the group Jalisa entered was very small, and all male; one male was Latino. Also by chance, those males were encouraging and nurturing without being domineering. Remember the story I told about Richard Katz running with the Kalahari K'ung? This was the same. The male group members encouraged her, they didn't slow down in playing the song, but their encouragement and unspoken expectation that she was capable of playing her part was magical and healing. Jalisa began to play with far greater confidence and accuracy; her sense of rhythm was excellent once she began to play, as she said, *con gana* (with enthusiasm, with passion). The drumming became celebratory in this small group as the progress in personal healing was evident. I most remember the last time this small group played together, Jalisa book-ended by males on either side, her in the center, all smiling and playing "con gana".

CHAPTER 7

Therapeutic interventions part II: treating mood disorders

"A village without music is a dead place." ~ *African proverb* (Hart, 1990, p. 195).

For readers who are unfamiliar with mood disorders, a brief overview is provided here. More thorough information is abundantly available from the websites of the National Institutes for Mental Health (NIMH), the Diagnostic and Statistical Manual of Mental Disorders 5th edition (DSM-5), as well as numerous articles and books on these disorders.

The category, "mood disorders," encompasses roughly 19 separate disorders. These can be grouped in three major categories: depressive disorders, anxiety disorders, and bipolar disorders. The hallmark of depressive disorders is extreme sadness, hopelessness, lack of energy, low motivation, changes in appetite and sleep (either too much or too little), and withdrawal from the activities that the individual used to find pleasurable. There are often gender differences in how depression appears. Depressed women are more likely to weep, while depressed men may not cry but instead show irritability and anger. It is important for therapists to distinguish between an underlying depression, or a problem with anger management. Depression can lead to suicide, so it is important for a therapist to ensure that the individual is not actively suicidal, or to take steps to ensure that they will be prevented from making an attempt.

Bipolar disorder includes episodes of depression, but it also includes marked increases in goal-directed behavior with little need for sleep. This latter part of the bipolar cycle is called mania. When an individual is manic, they have boundless energy, need little sleep, and tend to engage in risky behaviors that seem like a good idea at the time, like engaging in sex with multiple partners without protection, or charging the credit card to the max, or heavy drinking or drugging. The negative outcomes associated with risky behaviors tend to exacerbate the individual's descent into depression, as they find themselves dealing with huge bills, sexually transmitted diseases, or a DUI arrest. Some individuals have cycles of depression and hypomanic episodes, meaning that their mania is not quite so extreme, but they still might get themselves in trouble. It is not unusual for the person with a bipolar disorder to have lost employment and to have left significant relationships in chaos and confusion. Bipolar disorder is not unlike a roller-coaster ride, up and down, with the effects felt not only by the individual with the disorder, but by persons close to that individual.

Anxiety disorders represent an individual's fears and fear-based behaviors. These fears are typically exaggerated or unrealistic; for example, driving on the freeway is indeed dangerous, but you are unlikely to be killed when you get in the car to drive to work. The shopping mall is indeed filled with strangers, but it is unlikely that they are going to laugh at you or insult you publicly. Yes, there are bacteria and viruses all around us, but washing your hands 50 times a day will dry and crack the skin on your hands, exposing you to a greater likelihood of an infection. Panic attacks are experienced by a good portion of persons with anxiety disorders. Sometimes an individual is fearful and worries constantly, without knowing exactly what they are worried about. Unfortunately, unrelenting fear affects more than the brain; the body gets flooded with a chemical called cortisol, which can cause damage to internal organs over time. Significant sleep problems are very common in persons with anxiety disorders, and sleep medications are often addictive.

As with the clients whose primary diagnosis is a substance use disorder, here as well there are often co-occurring disorders. It is not unusual for an individual with an anxiety disorder, for example, to also have a personality disorder. By definition, a personality disorder is "an enduring pattern of inner experience and behavior that deviates markedly from the expectations of the individual's culture, is pervasive and inflexible, is stable over time, and leads to distress or impairment" (DSM, p. 645). There are eleven different personality disorders, with features that vary widely. Suffice it to say that an individual with personality disorders, even without a mood disorder, often has difficulty navigating the requirements of adult life, and/or causes disruption to the lives of those around them due to their associated behaviors. The combination of a mood disorder with a personality disorder generally indicates the need for longer-term treatment; often three to five years of at least weekly therapy sessions. In therapy, the anxiety, depression, or bipolar disorder is often tackled first and these are very amenable to treatment. The most effective treatment is a combination of medication and therapy.

Common areas of deficit

As described above, there are distinct features of each type of mood disorder, and some overlap, such as sleep disruption. Here is a list of some common problem areas we might find in persons with mood disorders:

- Emotional regulation; ie, managing one's emotions effectively
- Lack of energy, lack of motivation
- Hopelessness
- Fear of embarrassment, of making a mistake
- Fear of being judged negatively by peers
- Fears associated with specific triggers: lightning, snakes, germs, needles (to name a few)
- Low self-esteem
- Unrealistic ideals of relationships
- Cynical outlook on life
- Harsh self-judgment
- Self-defeating behaviors
- Perfectionism
- Thinking errors, dysfunctional "automatic thoughts"
- Unrealistic expectations of self
- Stuck in unsuccessful patterns of behavior
- Employment problems
- Financial difficulties
- Physical health issues
- Strained/broken relationships

Of course, this will vary from person to person and with the specific type of disorder. Each individual is unique and has a unique set of resources, inner and outer, that also impact how they deal with their depression or anxiety. Persons who come to treatment for these disorders typically have been unsuccessful in coping with their problematic thoughts, feelings, and behaviors. They need help repairing the major sectors of their life that have been affected: work/school, relationships, and personal well-being.

How traditional West-African drumming addresses areas of deficit

When a person's mental illness causes significant disruption in the major areas of functioning in his/her life, they come to us feeling very broken and defective. Their self-esteem is low, and there is a reluctance to try new ways of thinking, feeling, and acting. They may often mistrust others because others have rejected them or let them down before. Interpersonal functioning may be impaired. Thus, establishing a safe environment of trust and positive regard for clients is essential. Creating a high likelihood of early success, even a small achievement, is also important so the client has something to build on. Drumming allows this, as the basic drum strokes are quite simple despite being more difficult to perfect.

The brilliant Russian psychologist, Lev Vygotsky, found that learning occurs most effectively in the context of interpersonal interaction (1978). Further, he found that using a technique of *scaffolding* allows learners to experience a personal sense of possibility in learning. Scaffolding, as the word suggests, simply means a ladder-like sequence of small steps towards a goal. In drumming, we start with the basic three notes of bass, tone, slap, before attempting to learn parts to a song. Then we learn one djembe part. We introduce a second part, and then put together the two parts, or more. When drummers can play parts solidly together, we might increase the speed/pace. This is scaffolding in drumming.

Vygotsky conceptualized the *zone of proximal development* or ZPD. The ZPD concept has three components or possible positions relevant to teaching and learning: first, overshooting the learner's ability level; second, undershooting the learner's ability level; and third, finding the optimal target to stretch the learner by utilizing their current knowledge base and offering just a little bit more. In the first scenario, if you present the student with material they have already mastered, they will be bored and become disengaged. Conversely, if you present the learner with material that is way beyond their current mastery level, and thus too difficult for them to grasp, they will become frustrated and also disengage from the learning process. The optimal position in the ZPD uses the student's current knowledge base as a launch pad to reach for the next higher level. This might mean stretching their comfort zone, or simply a mental stretch. A good math teacher, for example, scaffolds the process from the simple (addition and subtraction) to more complex processes (long division, multiplication) before tackling quadratic equations. The teacher who broaches the topic of fractions before allowing students to master simple numeracy skills will disenfranchise the students. Likewise, the teacher who teaches basic addition to calculus students is likely to lose them to obvious yawns.

So how do we apply this to drumming? Using the ZPD concepts, we introduce new material little by little, and build upon each small increase in mastery. I can't expect a new drummer to perform a 4-stroke roll when they might still be afraid to strike the drum. The bass is the simplest stroke to execute correctly; it makes a satisfying, resonant sound. And we build from there. In terms of interpersonal dynamics, I watch the clients carefully to identify the level of their current interpersonal skills. Some mood-disordered clients are highly guarded and avoid interaction. Some are highly anxious and project that with nervous laughter and excessive chatter. Some sit slumped with eyes downcast.

The famous Viennese psychiatrist, Alfred Adler (1998), said that one of the major human problems is discouragement. He wrote it like this: dis-couragement. Meaning, we lose our courage. In order to recover from discouragement, we need to be en-couraged; in other words, to regain our courage. I share this idea with my clients; I am transparent in my encouragement but do not shower them with empty reassurances nor gratuitous praise. I see them trying, and praise their effort. I hear them make a pleasing sound on the drum, and I praise that. I see their fear of trying a step that is a bit more difficult, and I encourage them to stretch their comfort zone. Little by little, their engagement increases as they feel they are on solid ground with their basic drumming skills. Because I've modeled encouragement, they begin to praise each other and make encouraging statements to each other. I make space in the group for this to occur. Example:

Bridget: *quietly crying in her seat, drum between her knees*
Me: Bridget, what are the tears about?
Bridget: I can't get it!
Me: You can't get what?
Bridget: I can't play the part!
Me: What seems to be getting in the way?
Bridget: I don't know. I just can't do it.
Me: Has anyone else in the group felt this way? Tell Bridget.
Mary: Bridget, it was like that for me when I first started, too. I didn't think I could get it, but I just kept trying, and it seemed to click after about the third time.
Me: Bridget, how does it feel to hear about Mary's experience?
Bridget: That's good for her.
Delphinia: I actually think you're doing fine, Bridget. Maybe better than you think you are. Just give yourself a chance.
Bridget: (sighs) I know, I know, I'm always too hard on myself.

One other approach I use is more physical than mental, but the two blend in this exercise. *Triplets* in drumming are as the name suggests; a rhythmic pattern consisting of three notes played by alternating hands and in equal timing: 1-2-3. Bass-tone-tone or Bass-slap-slap. This is a djembe part for a number of different traditional West-African songs, but I use it as a practice drill. I start with the clients playing very slowly, 1-2-3-1-2-3 and so on. We might pick up the speed a bit to stretch their ability level. Then we start over again, with chairs side-by-side close together so that each person can reach over and play a bass stroke on the person's djembe on either side of them. So for each bass note, every individual is reaching first to the right to play on the djembe of the person to their right, and then two tones on their own djembe, then reaching to the left to play a bass note on the djembe of the person to their left, then back to their own drum again for two tones. So as I play with them I say out loud: "REACH tone tone REACH tone tone" and so forth. What happens is a synchronization of movement, the clients' bodies swaying right and left with each "reach". Clients who might have difficulty with rhythm and coordination get pulled along with the swaying and the beat, and tend to do better rhythmically in this exercise than they would playing individually. Consistently I see more smiling and laughing in this drill than any other.

This exercise is especially effective with my female mood-disorder clients, many of whom have been emotionally wounded by other females and thus don't trust their female peers. It becomes a bonding experience, where the give-and-take of the body movement in drumming appears to create emotional space for mutual reliance, interdependence, and trust to begin germinating. It also represents an example of what we call "entrainment." Much has been written about entrainment in music and movement. "If two rhythms are nearly the same, and their sources are in close proximity, they will always entrain. Why? The best theory is that nature is efficient and it takes less energy to pulse together than in opposition" (Hart, 1990 p. 121). In this exercise, our natural tendency to move and play synchronistically aids in our emotional synchronicity as well.

Case histories

Case 1: Collette

Collette, age 29, came to treatment with an eating disorder, bipolar disorder, frequent panic attacks, and a personality disorder. She had been in treatment multiple times for her eating disorder and believed that was under control; it was not. She was newly diagnosed with bipolar disorder and required education on bipolar disorder and how to manage it. Many times individuals with bipolar disorder undergo a shift in identity, struggling to see themselves as a person with an illness that will require taking medication and developing coping strategies for their entire life. The adjustment is often extremely difficult, and these individuals very often stop taking their mood-stabilizing medication when they begin to feel better, thus throwing themselves into another cycle of depression and mania.

Initially Collette refused to participate in the drumming group; she was highly perfectionistic and if she couldn't excel immediately at something, she would not even try it. So, she was allowed to dance for the drummers, which she enjoyed. She would run and skip around the room, waving her arms in the air, laughing and sometimes crying out of a sheer confusion of emotions. Little by little, as she heard the drumming instruction and saw her peers begin to make small improvements, she would sit for a bit and give it a try.

She would quickly become frustrated with her lack of skill, and would quit drumming, at which point she would be directed to either "drum or dance," since leaving the group was not an option.

Since we drum as we live our lives, I asked Collette in the group what she was so afraid of? She was able, with the support and encouragement of her peers, to begin to explore and then articulate the source of her perfectionism: as a child she was scolded for making mistakes and felt humiliated and defective. Adding insult to injury, she also had abusive coaches in her adolescent sports years who berated her for being too slow, too heavy, a burden to the team. (She was none of these things.) She equated her value as a human being with her ability to excel at academics and sports. Collette understandably stuck with the skill sets she already possessed; anything else felt like a threat, throwing her into anxiety and depression. I encouraged her to b-r-e-a-t-h-e as she typically held her breath while drumming. As she gained insight through these conversations, both in group and in individual sessions, she was able to relax her body while drumming and increase her level of emotional engagement, with less fear of failure. She was able to state, near the end of her treatment, "I did my best. I made some mistakes, but that didn't matter."

Case 2: Mark

Mark, age 35, was an individual who had recently suffered a major depressive episode in which he attempted to end his life. He had lived for many years with dysthmia, a low-level depression that probably started in childhood. He lived with an alcoholic mother and his father had left the family when Mark was 15. Mark had not explored these family issues in a meaningful way prior to coming to treatment; one could fairly said that Mark was in denial about many aspects of his inner and outer life.

Mark had owned a very lucrative business in California; he had some public notoriety for his success and related media appearances. However, he had lost everything due to his abuse of benzodiazepines (anxiety-control medications). He took money from the business, and time, to use drugs. His professional reputation was significantly damaged when the business failed. His love life consisted primarily of a succession of women who were using drugs, and abusing him financially and emotionally, sometimes even physically. He would leave a woman, feel guilty, and return out of loyalty even when love was absent. This cycle never ended well. Mark would get clean (ie, stop using) for a period of time after giving himself a talking-to, but ultimately he always returned to using. His mother had been funding his apartment, but due to her own employment challenges, she stopped doing so and he moved in with mom in light of a lack of other options. This time, Mark had been clean from drugs for over a month, but his depression was crushing, he had suicidal thoughts, and he knew he needed help for this or he would return to using and, much as he loved his mother, he didn't want to live with her forever.

Mark was one of the rare clients I had in group who had drummed before. He had attended drum circles, and mimicked some videos on line of African drumming. His self-discipline was at a low level, and he was saturated in shame for his addiction, his attempt at suicide, loss of his business, and for living at home with his mother. His eye contact with me and with his peers initially consisted of furtive glances. He looked like a forlorn puppy who wants to be loved but expects to be kicked. He demonstrated some impatience with the elementary level of the drumming, but quickly developed empathy as he understood where his peers were coming from, which was very entry level. His prior experience, although not deep, allowed him to be seen as a leader, and he enjoyed this role. I encouraged his leadership as he brought a good deal of humility along with it.

As Mark made progress in individual therapy with his inner demons, and in family therapy with his mother, he became less defensive, softer, more relaxed in drumming. He became more altruistic with others as he began forgiving himself for mistakes of the past. He became a key encourager for group members who were struggling. Mark reserved his harshest judgments for himself, but as time went on he did less of that and found his drumming improving significantly. He could play a part solidly and consistently, and was proud of his inventive solos. He often smiled while drumming and even laughed, and made solid eye contact with everyone. While he had lacked assertiveness in the past and saw assertive statements as "too aggressive" for him, Mark began to practice appropriate self-advocacy with peers who tended to manipulate him. His historic lack of boundaries with his mother and with exploitative females was explored, and he began to build healthy boundaries. He demonstrated this in the group as well, even in such small factors as claiming a particular djembe for the session and not giving up a seat to someone else who preferred a particular location in the room. Where he had been a pushover who resented others' boundary violations, Mark became quietly assertive about his rights and the rights of others in the group.

Mark began to see the link between his lack of self-discipline in drumming and the failure of his business, where he had given himself too many breaks, financial and otherwise. He saw how he had let down the employees, who all lost their jobs due to his lack of attention and diligence. We were able to talk about his value for loyalty, and how he could bring that back to his relationships with anyone he chose, specifically those who earned his loyalty. He began to see the value of focused and sustained attention to a task, and how such dedication had positive outcomes not just in drumming, but in his interpersonal relationships. He began talking of plans to re-launch his business, and developed optimism for the future. He hoped to continue drumming after treatment, and sought my advice on purchasing a djembe.

CHAPTER 8

Therapeutic interventions part III: recovery from trauma/abuse

> "This will be our reply to violence: to make music more intensely, more beautifully, more devotedly than ever before." ~Leonard Bernstein

Trauma occurs when an individual is exposed to a situation in which death appears imminent, either to the individual, to a loved one, or even as a witness to severe interpersonal violence where the individual doesn't know the victim of that violence. This can take many forms. The stereotypical trauma survivor is a veteran of war who witnessed, was directly affected by, and/or took part in extreme violence. Persons who were physically abused in childhood may develop trauma disorders. Additionally, survivors of sexual assault experience detrimental results that extend well beyond their physical injuries. Obviously, it is important to be sure that a trauma survivor's physical injuries have been addressed appropriately. Continuing physical reminders, such as migraine headaches, are not unusual in this population.

One of the most intriguing questions in psychology is why two similar persons can be subjected to the same violent event, and one will suffer from a trauma disorder while the other will not. This ability to emerge relatively unscathed from traumatic events is generally called *resilience* (6 Risk Factors, 1994). Research on resilience reveals that individuals have certain "protective factors" that buffer them and allow them to bounce back more quickly from trauma and with less residual effects than others who have few protective factors. For example, having a strong connection with family and friends tends to prolong life and enhances physical health and emotional well-being. So interpersonal connection is a protective factor. Likewise, having a strong spiritual belief and/or participation in a community of like-minded spiritual people is also a protective factor. A belief that one has significant control over one's outcomes is also protective; that is, if I believe that by working hard I can earn a nice income, that is positive self-efficacy. On the other hand, if I believe that my outcomes are random and nothing I do will change that, I have low self-efficacy. The underlying variable is a sense of control in one's life. Often trauma survivors have the sense that they don't have much control over their outcomes, so their efforts may be random, episodic, and ineffective. Therapy can help with that.

Survivors of childhood sexual abuse tend to have better outcomes when they are able to tell someone about the abuse, and the abuse stops. They feel safe and secure, and believed. Individuals who tell a trusted person that they are being abused, and nothing is done to stop it, and/or they are not believed, and thus the abuse continues, tend to have the most negative outcomes, even in adulthood. Similarly, other victims of trauma such as combat veterans do better when they don't have to return to combat situations where they will be re-traumatized.

Common areas of deficit

Across various trauma-related diagnoses, we typically see the following symptoms develop due to the occurrence of an extreme stressor(s):

- Difficulty concentrating
- Memory problems (can't recall)
- Intrusive memories (recall things you don't want to remember)
- Unrelenting anxiety, expecting bad things to happen
- Startle response to sensory stimuli (ex: jumping when someone touches your shoulder)
- Sensitivity to light, sound
- Nervous behaviors (difficulty sitting still)
- Limited positive affect
- Skepticism in abundance
- Avoidance of new experiences, locations (ie, risk averse)
- Irritability and angry outbursts
- Hyper-vigilance (ie, constantly monitoring the situation, observing others excessively)
- Difficulty trusting others
- Loss of a sense of humor, inability to "play"

These symptoms often cause dysfunction in a person's life in major areas such as work or school, interpersonal relationships, and self-care. Co-occurring substance abuse is common in this population, but should not be assumed; thorough evaluation upon intake is essential.

How traditional West-African drumming addresses areas of deficit

As the prior two sections have demonstrated, traditional West-African drumming requires a certain level of self-control and self-discipline. But first, the facilitator must make significant efforts to create a safe environment. With survivors of trauma, I find that it is important to position the drummers so that they can see the door. Putting them in a situation where they can't see who might be entering behind them will exacerbate their already-existing hyper-vigilance and you will see a lot of rubber-necking as they overreact to every sound and movement.

As previously noted, loud sounds, especially on the drum, may provoke a startle reaction, so this must be addressed early on. We might decide, as a group, to play more softly if there is someone in the group whose trauma included gunfire or explosions. We might decide to put a small hand-towel over the drumhead, so that all our strokes are muffled. I find that asking group members if there are logistical or mechanical variables like this that we could change to better enable their full presence invites better participation as they see that I recognize and acknowledge the reality of their symptoms. Often they have less empathetic people in their lives who say, "You're safe now, what's the problem?" Traumatized individuals get the message that they should be fine, but they are far from fine. They may decide that it's better to suffer in silence and pretend they're alright.

I convened a group of women survivors of sexual abuse in a novel location, and at their request, we used low lighting. Using the aforementioned components of setting up a circle and being mindful of body position in relation to doors, we also spoke in soft tones. The lighting is especially important for persons whose trauma is recent; sensitivity to bright lights, especially fluorescents, is common.

In drumming with a trauma group, I might start with a reminder about mindful breathing, being present in this moment, with this group of people, in a healing activity. This is an opportunity to step away from past history and the burdens we carry. I communicate explicitly that this is a safe place to take a risk and try something new. If new drummers are willing to take the risk of trying something new, with zero chance for failure (because mistakes are expected and allowed), and no penalty for memory problems, there is a high likelihood of success. I invite peers to share with new drummers what it was like for them when they first started; this typically invites a recollection of fears of failure, anxiety, frustration, even anger. These feelings are validated, and the drummer with even a week of experience is likely to also talk about how they transcended those negative emotions and began reaping the benefits of drumming. Trust begins to build with peers when even one person gives voice to fears and frustrations. It opens up space for hope and a belief in personal progress towards healing.

Watch for the emergence of anger. Therapists look for *microexpressions* to determine an individual's inner emotional state, regardless of what the person states they are thinking or feeling (because some have been punished for their anger, or taught that it is wrong or bad). The client's face and body language give them away. Persons who are simmering with anger show it in their eyes, around their mouth, the jaw area, and in other places on the body. Psychologist Paul Ekman, well known for his studies of microexpressions, has an on-line training program to assist new therapists with learning these minute clues [see reference list for Ekman's website].

The emergence of anger is not a bad thing necessarily. It is not unusual for clients to have buried their anger for so long that they don't recognize its existence. For example, the client who was raped by a family member may begin to uncover her anger at the perpetrator, a burning resentment that was previously disallowed. Depression may mask that deep fury. Attempting to drum for the first time, or to learn a new part, creates frustration, and that often opens the door for repressed anger to find oxygen. Individual therapy may also have worked its magic in allowing the anger to be recognized and named. The facilitator may draw attention to signs of frustration and anger so it can be reflectively addressed in a healthy manner. Explosive anger will not be healthy for the individual nor the group. But just as hitting a tennis ball with energy can release some of that anger, so can hitting a drum. It allows the client to see that they can control the degree of energy directed at the drum and the manner in which they strike it; they are not out of control. They are managing that raging fire in a productive way.

For new drummers, repitition is key. The same small musical phrases are presented over and over, and the drummer hears the sounds reproduced all around them. The arm and hand movements likewise are repeated over and over; the body begins to remember the movements. Moments of focus increase when vigilance decreases, and vigilance decreases with relaxed effort.

For trauma survivors, establishing the meaning-making inherent in traditional West-African drumming is important. It's not just a musical activity, not a noise-making distraction, it is participation in a coherent cultural tradition that includes everyone in some way. All contributions to this meaning-making are valued: the role of playing a solid djembe part, the role of a listener, the role of a soloist, the role of a dancer, and the role of the encouraging and appreciative audience. Positivity is accentuated as community is built.

There is value in the structure of a song with a beginning and an end. The song starts with "the call," as discussed earlier. The call signals that we are all about to start playing this particular song. We begin together and play until the lead drummer plays the call again, otherwise known as "the break," which signals that we're going to end the song, and we all stop together. Trauma survivors live with a good deal of internal chaos, so the firm structure of the song, and within each song, the specific parts, provides predictability and grounding. Within that predictable structure there is room for surprises; specifically the kind of good surprise that arises when someone plays a melifluous solo, when peers' skills show distinct improvement that is heard around the group, or when drummers see each other smiling in enjoyment of the polyrhythmic music being produced in the *now*.

Case histories

Case 1: Carrie

Carrie was a young woman with green and purple hair and various tattoos and body piercings. She was visually noticeable. Conversely, she tended to be very quiet and seemed to try to make herself invisible, sitting off to the side in any group. She was unlikely to volunteer anything unless specifically called upon to speak. She was timid and always looked sad.

Carrie was a survivor of multiple childhood sexual assaults. After her parents divorced, her single mom was working many hours to make ends meet and so Carrie was a latchkey child. Sometimes her grandma would watch her after school, but many times after school Carrie came home to a cold and lonely house. One day, a neighborhood teenage boy she knew from the school bus stopped by after school to play games with her. He was kind to her, and she appreciated the attention that she had been craving. Slowly the nature of his attention changed and this 7-year-old found herself the victim of sexual abuse. The abuse continued for a few months; she didn't want to tell her mom because she was a sensitive child and knew how hard her mom was working and didn't want to burden her.

Mom and Carrie moved to a different neighborhood, but mom was still working a lot, now at two jobs, and Carrie, now age 12, once again was left alone. She made a friend, Marcy, who often visited her uncle next door. Carrie had many fun times with Marcy and soon felt welcome to come and go from that house. In therapy circles we would call this period of time "cultivation," as Marcy's uncle was grooming Carrie for future sexual exploitation. He abused Carrie sexually for several weeks until Carrie did tell her mother. The uncle was arrested, found guilty of child sexual abuse, and put in prison. Unfortunately for sexual abuse survivors, the emotional pain does not end when the abuse ends. Carrie had been suffering for over a decade with flashbacks, and difficulty with forming healthy boundaries. She struggled to end a relationship with an abusive boyfriend. Like all of us, she just wanted to be loved; she played a submissive role hoping someone would love her the right way.

Carrie desperately needed to cultivate assertiveness skills, and to address her self-imposed isolation in treatment, and her depression and anxiety. Much of this, of course, needed to be done in individual therapy sessions, and also family therapy. We began in drumming with getting her to focus on the present moment, and some body awareness since she had largely divorced herself from her bodily sensations. Simply striking her hand on the drum, gently at first, reminded her of the present moment; striking it hard stings a bit so it is difficult to ignore your body's presence in drumming.

Like Mark, described earlier, Carrie allowed her peers to be dominant with her, and she submissive. She would be figuratively pushed aside in the group; others' voices took center stage. She felt safer at the margins of the group. In working on her trauma history in individual sessions, she was finally able to tell her mother about her earliest abuse history, so that mom could be fully informed and become a more integral part of Carrie's healing process. This was a turning point, as Carrie stopped taking responsibility for how mom might feel burdened and allowed mom to feel whatever she was feeling. This opened up space for Carrie to focus on herself and to begin working through her multitude of feelings about her childhood trauma.

Over time, starting with a very tentative solo consisting of three bass notes and eyes staring blankly at the floor, we began to make progress with making Carrie's drum-voice heard. There were days when the old adage "two steps forward, one step back" was true for Carrie. It was difficult for her to sustain and tolerate her own visibility. As the djembe parts became more familiar and her comfort level with drumming increased, Carrie was more likely to step out with a slightly longer solo. When peers began encouraging her, she allowed moments of trust and belief. I won't say she blossomed, but the perfume of the bud was evident. I know that with further therapy she would indeed come into the fullness of that flower.

Case 2: John

John, at age 52, had been a first-responder for all his adult life. While he loved the work, and loved helping people, the nature of the work had taken a toll. John shared the many and varied things he had witnessed that shook him to his core: tragic traffic crashes, suicides, shootings, children drowned. As a first-responder, he was often first on the scene in the immediate aftermath of unimaginable horrors. As a first responder, it was typical that you don't express your emotions at work, and "you don't take that home with you to inflict on your family." In short, you just "push it down" and deal with it in silence. Over time, John began using alcohol to numb those feelings. A few beers after work with the guys turned into significant alcohol use, some health issues, and a DUI that could end his career. His wife was threatening to leave him, and she didn't understand what was going on. "He never talks to me."

For John, who loved people, he did trust his fellow officers and felt he could rely on them. He trusted his wife and family, who he characterized as "the best people on earth." The person he couldn't trust, was himself. He felt like he was "a ticking time bomb" and that it was just a matter of time before he exploded. He lived in daily fear that he would lose his mind, his job, and everything he held dear. The daily dose of trauma and tragedy had become more than he could stand. He hated himself for drinking, but he had no idea of what else to do to stop the pain. His sleep was very disrupted with nightmares of blood, carnage, and dead children. Even awake, he had flashbacks of dismembered bodies that twisted his stomach and tortured his mind. John said, "I am a broken man." He felt hopeless.

One of the great things that happened for John is that as soon as he arrived at the treatment center, he began receiving letters and phone calls from his pals on the force. These told him what a good man he was, and how much they valued him. This encouragement was priceless in John's willingness to open up in treatment. He received loving cards from family members, including his wife and sons, saying how they wanted their "old" husband/dad back. John wanted that too. I cautioned John, as I have many other clients, *not* to want the "old you" back. The old you was defective and lacked coping skills. The old you helped you slide into this state of brokenness.

What you want is to keep all the good aspects of you; but this crisis in your life, and the aftermath, is full of important learnings that will be valuable to you in the future. So don't throw the baby out with the bathwater, as the old saying goes. Embedded in our history and our failures and our mistakes are important lessons that we don't want to lose. That wisdom is hard-earned and will serve us well going forward.

John was good-naturedly uninterested in learning traditional West-African drumming or any other kind of music. His attention was inconsistent and yet the positive environment of drumming group allowed him to relax and begin a slow recovery of his sense of humor, a key sign of healing. John's humor was generally directed at me, as facilitator, as I was obviously a safe, non-defensive target and I typically mentioned it when I made drumming mistakes, as part of role-modeling that it's ok to make mistakes. His joking was never mean-spirited and it was clear he was testing the waters to see if it felt safe to laugh again. In individual sessions, he shared that he felt guilty enjoying life when so many people had suffered horrible tragedies (that he had seen personally). I told him what Samuel Johnson, a contemporary of Benjamin Franklin, had said long ago: "All the animals but man know that the principle task of life is to *enjoy it*." In other words, yes, it's alright to smile, laugh, enjoy. Clinging to a somber mood does not alleviate anyone's suffering.

CHAPTER 9

Therapeutic interventions part IV: youth at risk

"When God had made The Man, he made him out of stuff that sung all the time and glittered all over. Some angels got jealous and chopped him into millions of pieces, but still He glittered and hummed. So they beat Him down to nothing but sparks but each little spark had a shine and a song. So they covered each one over with mud. And the lonesomeness in the sparks made them hunt for one another, but the mud is deaf and dumb. Like all the other tumbling mud-balls, Janie had tried to show her shine." ~ Zora Neal Hurston, *Their Eyes Were Watching God*

Kouyate's (1994) film, *Keita*, shows the supernatural calling of the master griot (jeliba) to teach a boy, Mabo, the meaning of his name – the history of his culture culminating in his birth. This includes the legend of Sundjata; a key component of oral tradition in Mali, Africa. The story of the boy's ancestors includes history, myth, spirituality, and prophecy. In the story, Sundjata is a disabled child of royalty who is unjustly treated as an outcast, but grows in strength, wisdom, and magic to fulfill his destiny as a leader of his people. The film also conveys the friction between African tradition and mythology and the increasingly Westernized lifestyle and beliefs of today's Malian citizens. The transmission of culture is often lacking in today's urban Black youth, and drumming empowers them to retake their rightful roles as the next generation to transmit a proud cultural history to their children.

I volunteered for two summers to teach traditional West-African drumming to youth at risk through the Fort Myers (Florida) African-Carribean-American (AFCAAM) enrichment program. Through a grant to my employer, a local University, we were able to purchase ten djembes and a set of dunduns. Youth participants ranged in age from 9 to 19. All came from economically disadvantaged backgrounds, all were students of color, all were in under-performing urban schools. Most had one parent either in prison or addicted to drugs or both. All came to AFCAAM primarily to work on academic deficits.

Common areas of deficit

It was obvious from my initial meetings with the students that self-esteem was often lacking, and for many there was some degree of isolation and marginalization due to problems at home (for those who had a home). Individual self-discipline was inconsistent. Some of the students appeared to be depressed, and some had unresolved grief and loss issues due to untimely deaths of friends or family members, or the absence of a parent from the home (typically due to prison time, sometimes due to drug use). Undiagnosed learning disabilities were not uncommon, with attention deficits and hyperactivity present. Other challenges included: concentration/focus, listening skills, communication skills, delayed gratification, frustration tolerance, regulation of anxiety and other emotions, and general social skills. All of these, of course, are important for success in school, work, and relationships. Despite multiple risk factors, there were often protective factors such as good interpersonal bonds with select peers, siblings, and with staff at the AFCAAM program who provided mentoring and a sense of normalcy and structure. A few older students were patient and able to follow directions and show respect for teachers and peers. The program was also disciplined, with clear rules for participation. Positive older peers were recognized as role models for younger students. As often as sibling rivalry appeared, other times the bonds between siblings were strong and supportive.

Using African drumming to address some of the areas of deficit with youth at risk is not completely new. Bittman, Dickson, and Coddington (2009) examined the use of creative music-making in working with youth in juvenile justice residential facilities. They make the point that obstacles to effectively rehabilitate inner-city adolescents in staff-secure residential treatment centers should not be underestimated. Effective evidence-based protocols are lacking to help juveniles who are often angry, detached, frustrated, and in direct conflict with their peers. Facing a myriad of issues ranging from delinquency offenses to trauma, abuse, drug/alcohol use, peer pressure/gang-related activities, lack of structure in home environments, mental health diagnoses, and cognitive functioning difficulties, these adolescents present extraordinary challenges to an over-stressed juvenile justice system.

Similarly, the youth in the AFCAAM program encountered obstacles on a daily basis: racism and prejudice in the community, disrupted family systems, under-resourced schools, stressors related to food- and housing-insecurity. In short, they were dealing with some major concerns in their young lives that were beyond their ability to effectively address, and these concerns should not be underrated. Teaching them traditional West-African drumming was not going to erase these basic survival concerns, but it could help ameliorate some of the other individual behavioral and attitudinal challenges that would otherwise negatively impact their success in school and beyond.

Halperin et.al. (2012) studied the use of games and physical exercises to address some of the deficit areas of children with ADHD. The intent was to target underlying brain physiology through scaffolding; that is, to introduce challenge in levels just beyond the participant's current skills such that they will stretch with effort to the new level, but not so difficult that the challenge simply creates frustration. The Halperin study showed results persisting beyond the end of the intervention. These results included improvements in memory and focus, as well as behavioral improvements.

Other researchers have examined the use of "play" in helping children to improve both cognitive and social skills. Oren (2008) discussed children's preference for play versus talk therapy for the obvious reasons that play is "fun" and also that talk therapy requires verbal abilities that are underdeveloped in children. Specifically, talking about thoughts and feelings may be difficult and many children lack an adequate vocabulary for accurately stating what they are experiencing. Board games provide the fun factor, but also provide a venue for children to demonstrate their coping skills for dealing with the frustrations that naturally occur in competitive games. Emotional development can be observed and facilitated by the therapist as the game proceeds, and pro-social skills encouraged. In drumming the element of competition is largely absent as there are no winners or losers in drumming for the community or group. However, some children bring a competitive spirit to learning a new song, to learn it more quickly than peers, or to play faster and more accurately.

Streng (2008) worked with children recovering from trauma and/or bereavement using a "game" approach. A primary need in such work is to provide a sense of safety, and Streng found that providing structure to children provides that sense of safety. Thus, difficult thoughts, feelings, and behaviors can be productively addressed within that safe space. Streng found that, in addition to learning new behaviors, children gained skill in interpersonal interaction and developed helpful insight into their own difficulties.

I established three drumming groups for instruction, as I wanted to establish a small "community" experience but also wanted to be able to give personal attention to each student. I clustered the students by age, as attention span tends to increase with age and I knew I would need to teach the youngest students in shorter segments. Each group had roughly 10 participants. All groups received instruction in the basics, as none of them had ever played the djembe before.

Sadly, as schools in the United States provide little or no exposure to the history or culture of the African continent, the pupils knew nothing about their African (and mixed) heritage or the role of traditional West-African drumming in Africa. Participatory socialization is a critical factor in the development of an aesthetic musical tradition (Harrison, in Jackson ed., 1985); this would include appreciation for the rituals, religious beliefs, or other aspects of the culture that form integral interplay in this music. For example, I asked the students, "How many countries are in Africa?" The answers ranged from "three" to "17." "There are actually 54," I replied, a fact which resulted in gasps of surprise. I shared a little bit about colonialism; why, for example, Africans in countries like Guinea speak French, and why the French were there in the first place. I shared about indigenous religions in West Africa, and what happened when the Europeans brought Christianity to Africa. I provided these informational moments in short segments so that each lesson focused on drumming but gave a bit of context and value. I wanted the students to value the history of their ancestors as a foil to the daily racism they experience in south Florida.

Each of the three groups learned a unique song so they could "show off" to their peers in other groups, knowing a song that others didn't know. They were taught the meaning of the song and why/when it would be played. They also knew that African drummers played for dancers, and that everyone else in the village would encourage and applaud the performers.

How traditional West-African drumming addresses areas of deficit

In addition to some of the key benefits of drumming described earlier, John Mews (2014) described additional gains to be found in working with children with special needs, such as impulse control and eye-hand coordination. Surprisingly, he found that the rhythmic drum sounds mimicked syllables and also helped students with sentence construction and other elements of communication. Increases in self-esteem and "fun" were reported.

Basic rules and requirements for participation in the AFCAAM program carried over to the drumming program. Students were expected to attend regularly (4 days per week) and punctually. They were subject to expectations for the academic components of AFCAAM and could not come just for drumming. Over 20 children signed up for the initial offering of traditional West-African drumming; these were organized into 3 groups. As mentioned previously, each group learned a specific song that they would perform for their peers at the end of the summer, thus fomenting the formation of community within each group. They learned not just the mechanics of the songs, but the meaning of the song and the context within which the song would be played in the traditional West-African village. Drumming requires a good deal of motor control; it also requires the ability to listen and follow directions. Learning a song with multiple parts requires memorization, focus, and patience; all skills that are important for success in school and interpersonal relationships.

I occasionally showed the students video clips of drumming and dancing in West Africa. I emphasized cooperation and communication as essential factors in learning to drum, as these are pro-social behaviors essential to successful work and relationships. They also had to listen to instructions, listen to each other, and be reliable and dependable in playing their parts. They were required to respect the instruments and treat them as the valuable artifacts that they are.

An important aspect of the education I shared with the students was my demonstration of respect for the peoples of Africa and the resilience they had shown over time in the face of Europeans strategically removing valuable resources from their lands and leaving little in return. The students developed respect for me, despite my Whiteness, and AFCAAM staff and parents alike voiced surprise that the children chose to give me authority over them in the drumming program. The literature on Racial Identity Development is relevant here (Ponterotto & Pedersen, 1998); the students were being provided with factual information about their heritage that countered prevailing myths in south Florida, where racism is rampant and discrimination saturates schools and neighborhoods. I saw the development of pride in students' Blackness.

I emphasized that this was an activity in which every person is important, valued, and interdependent. However, I did want to allow time for individual expression, so each person was invited to play a brief solo to say something unique to them on the drum. They were allowed to pass if they didn't care to solo, but most did. This not only underscored turn-taking behaviors and multitasking abilities, it provided a good balance between group focus and a brief moment to shine as an individual. Some worked to develop their solos for performance.

Another important aspect was FUN! Kids plus summer session can be drudgery, and it had to be fun. I told them that I wanted to have fun too, and it was most likely to be fun if everyone cooperated, if everyone encouraged each other instead of criticizing. They were skeptical, but I modeled this encouragement daily and we all did have fun and respect developed as each individual's drumming skill developed over the weeks. I also removed most of the pressure component; staff wanted the kids to perform for parents at the end of the summer. Using democratic process, I opened it up to the children to decide, and they did not want to perform for parents, so we didn't. Interestingly, in the second year of the program, the vote went the other way so we did perform for a larger audience.

Much to my surprise, several students from the first summer also signed up for the second summer. They were hooked on drumming. In fact, many of them progressed so rapidly that we were invited to perform at a few venues in the community, which was a huge boost to their self-esteem. I was told by staff the following year that one of the girls who thought she "wasn't musical" had decided to take up the flute in school, something her parents were thrilled about as she hadn't felt confident enough to sign up for music in school previously. The staff and parents attributed this increased confidence and willingness to take a risk to the girl's experience drumming with us in the prior two summers.

Another staff member from the university did some outcome interviewing with the students, asking them about their experience. Some responses were, "I felt like I was in Africa!" "I learned how to drum, and it was cool." "Our group got swag."

Case histories

There were many endearing students who took up residence in my heart and mind. I'll share the stories of two.

Case 1: Antonio

Antonio was in foster care in a family with young children, where he helped with childcare. Antonio had repeated a number of grade levels in school, so he was among the oldest in the program. He was a good athlete, but not good enough to get a college scholarship, so he was not college-bound. His biological father was in prison, and mother's location unknown. Antonio was not the best drummer. He struggled with learning the parts and with keeping tempo. His major asset was a positive attitude and a self-deprecating sense of humor. He was generous in his support of others and resisted any impulse to criticize peers. His attendance was consistent and it was clear that he always tried, even if his outcomes were not the best. He also had a quality of acceptance and tolerance, and clearly enjoyed connecting with others. Due to these qualities, he was accepted and appreciated by his peers. He modeled respect for staff and students alike. He was thoughtful and appreciative, and simply glowed when receiving positive attention.

Antonio was a reflective individual who was able to weigh the possible outcomes of his choices. At one point I offered to loan Antonio a drum to take home and practice, which otherwise was simply not done; and most would consider such an offer both a sign of respect and an honor, since the drums were so valuable and we treated them as sacred objects. He considered this offer, and then declined because he was concerned that the drum would be damaged by one of the younger children in the home. Antonio appeared to gain pride in his cultural heritage through the program; he sat a little straighter and stood taller.

Antonio appeared to understand his role as a supportive djembe player, not a soloist, and maintained that role; in other words, he both accepted and valued his place in this community of his peers. His sense of self-esteem grew as he recognized the respect he received from peers and facilitator. He was one of the students who returned in the second summer session of this program, and resumed his role. When I invited him to join a small performance group, he declined; he seemed to know his limitations and preferred to let his fellow drummers shine.

Case 2: Sha'rae

Sha'rae was a very slender teenager who appeared to have an untreated eating disorder. She initially gave me little to no eye contact, and when she did, it appeared as a glare, as if she were daring me to test her patience. Sha'rae had an initial diagnosis of ADHD which was later changed to Bipolar Disorder. Her energy would race, and thoughts would tumble out of her mouth without regard to the circumstance of time or place. She also had a history of abuse as a child, at the hands of particular family members. Some days she appeared to be grieving, withdrawn inside herself. She seemed to want to disappear into the chair or the floor. She seemed to feel safe when in the company of another girl in the group. My strategy was to allow her to be, and to encourage her to join in with the community formed by her particular group.

Little by little, Sha'rae began learning the parts. She listened to the mini-lectures on African culture with wide eyes and some apparent disbelief. She began to smile more, and participate more. Instead of her shoulders being up around her ears as a reflection of her experienced stress, or slumped when she was depressed, she appeared more relaxed with a neutral mood. She participated in the mini-competitions I set up between teams from the same group, to see who could play certain drills the fastest.

The single strategy that brought forth Sha'rae's confidence the most was when I invited her to play a part on the big drum, the dundun. I selected a simple rhythm and taught it to her individually before having her play with the group. We had established a norm of "everybody makes mistakes, just do it with style!" This helped give her permission to take the risk of doing something new and different where she would be more visible than she typically preferred. She played that part with energy and more assertiveness than I had seen in the prior weeks! Everyone in the group smiled and enjoyed this new Sha'rae who had suddenly emerged as a drum diva in the group. Where previously she had often been off the beat due to her hesitation, now she played more rhythmically and in consonance with her peers due to her ability to attack the notes with greater confidence. When I saw her again the next summer, she had gained some weight and her overall mood was much more even (also due to changes in medication) and her drumming greatly improved. She was able to immediately look me in the eye with a relaxed smile.

CHAPTER 10

Conclusion: Rock on with your Bad Self

> "There is a vitality, a life force, an energy, a quickening that is translated through you into action, and because there is only one of you in all time, this expression is unique." ~ Martha Graham

In my drumming experience in Brockport, New York, I took on an informal role as communicator-in-general for the group, to make the logistical end of things easier on our beloved drum master, Khalid Saleem. I would send out e-mails to the group about scheduling of practices, upcoming performances, cancellations and delays. In the group we joked frequently about old songs like "Ring My Bell" and lyrics like "Tighten Up!" One favorite was "Rock On With Your Bad Self." I began signing my emails to the group with this lyric, and eventually shortened it to "ROWYBS" and that stuck. I even made T-shirts with this and had my daughter create a djembe logo, which you see on the cover of this book. When times are tough –and there will always be tough times—the thought of my drumming community supporting and encouraging me through it allows me to tell myself: ROWYBS. Keep going! Smile while you do it! And this helps me to bounce back. I believe it is possible to entrain ourselves with this positive attitude, and the experience of traditional West-African drumming helps create that enduring collective and meaningful vibe in a way that a drum circle never will.

Community is an essential bonding ground for humans to love, live, grow, and thrive. Through the many stages of human development, we need a healthy place to be encouraged, supported, and sometimes guided to higher performance. Each individual is valued and appreciated in a healthy community. Benjamin Franklin said, "We must all hang together, or surely we will all hang separately." Our common humanity calls us together, and together we must stay despite our differences.

Psychologist Norm Kagan (1995) said that we all need love. It is part of the human condition. But there are four major fears that get

in our way. These fears are:
1. You will hurt me.
2. I will hurt you.
3. You will suffocate me.
4. I will suffocate you.

Particularly as adults, many of us have borne the bruises of love battles, in our families and other emotionally intimate relationships with friends and partners. We have been devastated or suffocated; we have crushed or suffocated others. We carry these heart-wounds with us, either as old scars or, as one client put it, "an open gash." Naturally, we are cautious about allowing ourselves to be vulnerable. We want so badly to seek love, but we don't want to be hurt again. It is an internal tug-of-war: the closeness we crave versus a safe distance. We either risk getting hurt, or suffer the pain of isolation and loneliness. It is no wonder that we struggle with these impossible choices!

In *African Music: A People's Art*, drummer Francis Bebey says of African drumming, "It is an art form that can and must communicate with people of all races and cultures and that should enjoy the ultimate fate of all great currents of human thought – to make its mark on the present and future, while bringing a new breath of life to all mankind" (1969, p. vi). In order to make that mark, Bebey argues that drumming must be accessible to people everywhere. It must be explained to them, to deepen their cultural understanding. Such a deep understanding, he says, will reveal "inner truth" and lead us to "the threshold of human happiness." This bold claim can be realized, if we only heed the call.

The use of traditional West-African drumming allows us to both establish a collective bond and to use that bond to defend against the wounds of daily living. The drumming community becomes a salve, a predictable cocoon, a buffer that aids in our building resilience to face the challenges of living in this century. The traditional West-African drumming group provides structure, opportunities for pro-social engagement, mentoring younger drummers, encouraging those with deficits. It helps us rise toward becoming our "best self," stretching our comfort zone to grow nearer to the possibility of our higher purpose. At a profound level of performance, participants/listeners "hear" a beat that is not there; the performance reaches a rhythmic metaphysical level as an understanding of the music emerges that cannot be heard by those unappreciative of the culture and aesthetic (Chernoff, 1979, p.155). It is a spiritual experience when that occurs.

Earlier I talked about the evaluation I used with my clients, and here I share some of their voices in response to the questions I asked about their experience drumming:

Question: What did I learn about myself in group today?

I have rhythm and soul

It's good to try new things

Drums are a good way for me to meditate

I'm depressed a little or a lot idk [I don't know]

I can still learn

I am patient and have more rhythm than I was beginning to think

I have been improving.

I have nervous energy. I got to express it in my solo.

Every instrument is different, just like every person is different; that's what makes the world beautiful.

When I focus on other people I lose focus on myself.

I need to slow down and not get so distracted by outside forces. I can drum better each week.

I'm getting better with time.

I need to focus more on what I need to do, not what I want to do.

I can't self-mutilate. I'm better than that.

I have been able to focus and stay present.

How serene and relaxing it was and everyone working together as one.

I am more centered and focused mentally, physically, and emotionally.

I am able to focus much more and not have racing thoughts.

Question: How can I apply what I learned today in group to me?

Find a good therapeutic outlet when stressed.

Give everything a chance.

Focus my feelings and thoughts instead of racing thoughts, anxiety.

Learn to cope with my energy.

Music is very therapeutic.

I can slow myself down and think of myself as a wound-up drum that needs to release my pent up energy.

Focus on me instead of focusing on others, and things will be alright.

I can learn to acknowledge that I feel in a rush, but choose to slow down just for today.

Slow down and look at what I need to do to better myself.

I can be creative and fun, if I slow myself down.

I am focused more.

I can slow down and just for today play the bass.

Not to be sluggish and stop bringing myself down.

I need to focus on myself more.

I can focus on "just for today" and stay present in my recovery.

Serenity and relaxation are a very important part of sobriety and I can relate that towards myself to be and stay sober.

Slowing down and not rushing in life.

If you find all of this terribly intriguing and probably useful, I hope you will take steps to implement this in your practice. If you're a therapist and not yet a drummer, or you're a drummer and not a therapist, how can you get started?

First, for non-therapists, you need to know that well-intentioned but untrained "counselors" can do damage to vulnerable populations. It is essential that you obtain training in therapeutic concepts and techniques, or optimally, to pursue the credentialing necessary to becoming a licensed therapist. If that is unrealistic, I recommend that you team up with a trained group facilitator; hopefully someone who drums or is willing to learn.

If you're a therapist who hasn't yet learned to drum, the number one rule is to find a good teacher. There are some masquerading as teachers who are not grounded in the history, technique, nor culture. Do your research, ask around. There are many communities, large and small, where good drumming teachers can be found. There are also some websites and events that might be helpful. For example, Wula Drum [website: wuladrum.com] has an annual retreat in the mountains outside of New York City where there are days of dancing and drumming with amazing teachers. There is an event called Paralounge [website: paralounge.net] that has multiple locations and dates each year, mostly in the south, where drumming classes are held and nightly "jam" sessions with drummers famous and new. There are music therapy conventions where drumming may be present. Wula Drum sells a library of instructional CDs and DVDs that break down the traditional songs into djembe and dundun parts. Khalid Saleem has his Percussion Discussion instructional CDs. There are a multitude of videos on Youtube that might help you get started, but nothing can replace the richness of a group drumming experience. It takes time to develop the skill and knowledge base, so patience is essential.

I started this book by sharing "the call" and offering traditional West-African drumming as a salve to the modern illness of disconnection and loneliness that plagues many individuals and particularly those with mental disorders. Back in 1905, the German sociologist Max Weber warned of an "unprecedented inner loneliness of the single individual" that accompanied the "spirit" of modern capitalism (as cited in Stephenson, 2017). In a capitalist society founded on competition, privatization, and small family units, collective joy—as opposed to individual happiness—signals both personal resilience and political rebellion. The very act of relishing in a shared connection is a triumph in a society that seeks to divide us. Let us join together in creating joy and denying the forces that would contain and silence us.

Thank you for reading, and please, today and every day …
ROWYBS!

Glossary of Relevant terms

Animism – based on the Latin word 'anima' meaning soul or spirit, this belief system ascribes a soul or spirit to all objects and beings, including rocks, trees, stars, the ocean. The sacred is in all things; everything has divinity in its essence.

Bass – one of the 3 main sounds made on the djembe; this is with the full palm of the hand striking the center of the drum making a resonant, deep sound.

Ben – to meet or greet; to be in tune

Bon Festival – short for Japanese 'Obon' and based on Buddhist-Confucian beliefs for hundreds of years, the 'Bon Odori' is a time for drumming and dancing to honor departed ancestors and their sacrifices, and to show appreciation to the ancestors and for favors received (such as bountiful harvest).

Dakini – the dakini is variously a drummer, a demon, a wise angel, a minor deity; the dakini appears to have originated in Tibetan Buddhism but is also seen in spiritual literature from India, China, and Japan.

Djembe (also 'jembe') – single-headed drum shaped like a goblet and played with both hands; it is widespread in eastern Senegal, Mali, Guinea, Burkina Faso, and Cote d'Ivoire (Ivory Coast). The drum is traditionally carved from a single piece of wood; the type of wood influences the sound, as does the size and shape. The drum head is typically made of goat skin; the thickness and type of skin also influences the sound.

Djembefola – people who play the drum

Dundun (also 'dunun' and 'dundunba') – large double-headed cylindrical drum played with a stick; sometimes refers to all types of such drums, typically refers to the largest of 3 double-headed drums with a deep bass sound.

Entrainment – pulse, memory storage, internal sense of periodicity, *feel* the relationships between beats, measuring accents of strong/weak beats, time/pause between phrases, qualitative recognition of sub-pulse rhythms (Iyer V.S., 1998, p. 33)

Ethnomusicology - "music as a universal aspect of human behavior" (Nketia, 2005, p. 21); study of music in culture; intersection of anthropology and music; quest for 'meaning' in music. Components: understanding what the musicians are doing, understanding the song, what the drums are saying, why the piece is being played, norms of behavior in musical situations, other things happening at the musical event that might be relevant.

Genki – a Japanese term meaning the source of vitality, a lively force; one with 'genki spirit' is lively and healthy, robust.

Griot – see 'jeli' below.

Jeli – an oral historian and musician; a hereditary role. The French colonists who came to Africa called this the *griot*.

Jelidon – the jeli people

Jelike – a male jeli

Jelimuso – a female jeli

Kenkeni – the smallest of the 3 dundun drums with a high-pitched sound.

Mnemonics - a code or cue to facilitate memorization or recall, often involving imagery or alliteration; "Rhythms are frequently represented as linguistically derived mnemonics, an obviously favored technique in an oral culture" (Iyer, 1998, p. 90).

Paramusic - feeling the vibration of the drums, seeing the dancers' footwork, observing the musicians' body language (Iyer, 1998 p. 86)

Polyrhythm – multiple rhythms appearing simultaneously; in African music cyclic rhythms are common (Iyer, 1998, p. 13) … "interlocking" rhythmic quality in African and African-American music (p. 15); includes a degree of 'animation' and spontaneity as relevant to the functional role of music in African and African-American communities (p. 16), an activity that is integral to life and everyday reality. Bell patterns assist in grouping drum patterns and orient listeners; "beat" is assumed in the mind of the listener and the musician but may not be apparent to Westerners. (Iyer, 1998, p 88)

Pulse - any periodicity inherent or perceived in any rhythm or combination of rhythms (Iyer, 1998, p. 12); roughly equivalent to 'beat'

Red Road – In Native American terms, an individual who attempts to live by the Creator's guidance and instructions is on the Red Road. Truth, humility, respect, and spirit are all part of this path. There is a distinction between being "on" the Red Road and "walking" the Red Road, the latter of which is a more rigorous and self-disciplined activity. [see website http://nacwr.blogspot.com/2011/07/walking-red-road.html]

Rhythm - any perceived or inferred temporal organization in a series of events (Iyer V.S., 1998, p. 12) – example: ocean waves, sewing machine

Sangban – the medium-sized dundun drum, often carries the melody.

Sensei – a Japanese term meaning "one who has gone before"; usually refers to an elder or teacher of a profession, often the martial arts.

Shinto – Japan's indigenous religion based on ancient peoples' fears of demons and spirits and rituals to appease the gods and receive favors (such as a bountiful harvest).

Shinto shrine – a sacred place where the kami (Gods) are worshipped; a place where the embodiment and integration of all things is represented symbolically.

Slap - one of the 3 main sounds made on the djembe; this is with the finger tips ricocheting off the head near the edge of the drum, making a high sharp sound

Sun Dance – "The name Sun Dance derives from the Sioux identification of it as *Wi wanyang wacipi*, translated as 'sun gazing dance'," according to the Encyclopedia of the Great Plains.

Originating with the Plains Indian nations, this sacred ceremony was suppressed for many years by both the US and Canadian governments as a superstition, so these dominant groups denied freedom of expression to the Original Nations. It was practiced in secrecy in some areas, while it died out in others due to the dominant groups' pejorative ideas about the practice. It began resurfacing more publicly in the mid 1900s as Native Americans reclaimed their right to practice their beliefs, and for its original purposes. According to the Encyclopedia of the Great Plains, the central concern of the Sun Dance is to establish and maintain kinship with all the people's relatives, including other humans, the animal and plant relatives of this earth, and the cosmic relatives of the spirit realm. To do so, sacrifices are made by participants, such as fasting, purification, and piercing of the skin as part of preparation and enactment of the ceremony. The Sun Dance lasts for several days. (Wishart, n.d.).

Turtle Island – the Original Nations referred to North America as Turtle Island, according to website Indian Country Today; some Native Americans refer to persons in the US and Canada as "living on Turtle Island." (Newcomb, n.d.).

Tempo - It is common in African music to accelerate the tempo; Western listeners may misinterpret this as an inability to maintain a steady pace (Chernoff, 1979, p. 97).

Tone - one of the 3 main sounds made on the djembe; this is with the fingers striking the drum head flatly near the rim

Umoja – Swahili word for unity; a state of being one or undivided. To strive for and to maintain unity in the family, community, nation.

Wadaiko – literally: large Japanese drum; also used to symbolically refer to the circle in a spiritual sense.

References

6 Risk and Protective Factors for the Onset of Mental Disorders. Institute of Medicine. 1994. *Reducing Risks for Mental Disorders: Frontiers for Preventive Intervention Research.* Washington, DC: The National Academies Press. Doi: 10.17226/2139.

Adler, A. as translated by Brett, C. (1998). Understanding Human Nature. Hazelden.

Akta Lakota Museum and Cultural Center. The Native American Drum. Retrieved July 15, 2017 from http://aktalakota.stjo.org/site/News2?page=NewsArticle&id=8913

American Music Therapy Association. Retrieved December 18, 2017 from https://www.musictherapy.org/about/requirements/

Ballinger, B. & Yalom, I. (1995). The theory and practice of group psychotherapy, 4th ed. New York: Basic Books.

Bebey, F. translated by Bennett, J. (1969). *African Music: A People's Art.* Brooklyn: Lawrence Hill Books.

Billmeier, U. and Keita, M. (1999). *A life for the djembe: Traditional rhythms of the Malinke.* Freiberg: Arun-Verlag.

Bittman, B., Berk, L., Felten, D.L., Westengard, J., Simonton, Pappas, and Ninehouser (2001). Composite effects of group drumming music therapy on modulation of neuroendocrine-immune parameters in normal subjects, *Alternative Therapies*, Vol. 7, No. 1.

Bittman, B., Berk, L., Shannon, M., Sharaf, M., Westengard, J., Guegler, K.J., and Ruff, D.W. (2005) Recreational music-making modulates the human stress response: a preliminary individualized gene expression strategy. *Medical science monitor : international medical journal of experimental and clinical research*, Vol.11(2), pp.BR31-40.

Bittman, Bruhn, K. T., Stevens, C., Westengard, J., and Umbach, P.O. (2003). Recreational music-making: a cost-effective group interdisciplinary strategy for reducing burnout and improving mood states in long-term care workers, *Advances in Mind-Body Medicine*, Fall/Winter 2003, Vol. 19 No. 3/4.

Bittman, B. , Dickson, L., Coddington, K. (2009) Creative musical expression as a catalyst for quality-of-life improvement in inner-city adolescents placed in a court-referred residential treatment program. *Advances in mind-body medicine*. Vol. 24, No. 1, p. 8-19.

Bittman, B., Croft, D.T., Brinker, J., Van Laar, R., Vernalis, M.N., Ellsworth, D.L. (2013). Recreational music-making alters gene expression pathways in patients with coronary heart disease. *Medical Science Monitor: International medical journal of experimental and clinical research*. 2013, Vol. 19, pp. 139-47.

Blum K[1], Schoenthaler SJ, Oscar-Berman M, Giordano J, Madigan MA, Braverman ER, Han D. (2014). Drug abuse relapse rates linked to level of education: can we repair hypodopaminergic-induced cognitive decline with nutrient therapy? *Phys Sportsmed.* 2014 May;42(2):130-45. doi: 10.3810/psm.2014.05.2065.

Bly, R. (1990). *Iron John: A Book About Men.* Addison: Reading MA.

Bolen, J.S. (1999). *The Millionth Circle: How to change ourselves and the world.* Berkeley, CA: Conari Press.

Brach, T. (2003). *Radical Acceptance: Embracing your life with the heart of a buddha.* New York: Bantam Books.

Burdette, J. (2017). Favorite music has greatest impact on brain connectivity. *News Medical Life Sciences.* Retrieved November 12, 2017, from https://www.news-medical.net/news/20170412/Favorite-music-has-greatest-impact-on-brain-connectivity.aspx

Caccioppo, J. et al (2007). Social Neuroscience: Progress and Implications for Mental Health. In: *Perspectives on psychological science*. Vol. 2, No. 2, p 99-101. Association for Psychological Science.

Center for Substance Abuse Treatment. *Substance Abuse Treatment: Group Therapy*. Treatment Improvement Protocol (TIP) Series, No.

41. HHS Publication No. (SMA) 15-3991. Rockville, MD: Substance Abuse and Mental Health Services Administration, 2005.

Charry, E. (2000). *Mande music: Traditional and modern music of the Maninka and Mandinka of western Africa*. Chicago: University of Chicago Press.

Chernoff, J.M. (1979) *African rhythm and African sensibility: Aesthetics and social action in African musical idioms*. Chicago: The University of Chicago Press.

Darwin, C. (1859). *On Origin of the Species*. NY: D. Appleton & Co.

DSM-5, *Diagnostic and Statistical Manual of Mental Disorders*, 5th ed. (2013). Washington DC: American Psychiatric Association.

Diallo, Y. and Hall, M. (1989). *The Healing Drum*: *African Wisdom Teachings*. Rochester, VT: Destiny Books.

DiClemente, C. (2003). *Addiction and change: How addictions develop and addicted people recover*. New York: Guilford Press.

Drake, Michael (2006). Therapeutic Effects of Drumming. Retrieved July 7, 2017, from https://www.scribd.com/document/28220586/Therapeutic-Effects-of-Drumming.

Ekman, P. (n.d.) *Microexpressions training tools*. Retrieved December 27, 2017, from https://www.paulekman.com/micro-expressions-training-tools/.

Frankl, V. (1959). *Man's Search for Meaning*. Boston: Beacon Press.

Gibran, K. (1926). *Sand and Foam*. New York: Alfred A. Knopf.

Harrison, D. (1985) Aesthetic and social aspects of music in African Ritual Settings. Pp. 49-66. In Jackson (ed) *More than drumming: Essays on African and Afro-Latin American music and musicians*. Westport, CT: Greenwood Press.

Halperin, J, Marks, D, Bedard, A, Chacko, A, Curchack J, Yoo, C, and Healey, D. (2012) Training executive, attention, and motor skills: a proof-of-concept study in preschool children with ADHD. In *Journal of Attention Disorders*, 17(8) 711–721. Sage Publications. DOI: 10.1177/1087054711435681

Hart, M. (1990). *Drumming at the edge of magic*. Harper SanFrancisco.

Hennig, H. & Fleischmann, R. & Geisel, T. (2012). Musical rhythms: The science of being slightly off. *Physics Today*. 65. 64-65. 10.1063/PT.3.1650.

Holt-Lunstad J, Smith TB, Layton JB (2010) Social Relationships and Mortality Risk: A Meta-analytic Review. PLoS Med7(7): e1000316. https://doi.org/10.1371/journal.pmed.1000316

Hyman, S. (2017). *Top 10 barriers to self-growth.* Dr. Stan Hyman Psychotherapy and Coaching. Retrieved November 28, 2017, from https://drstanhyman.com/top-10-barriers-to-self-growth/.

Iyer V.S. (1998). Microstructures of feel, macrostructures of sound: Embodied cognition in West African and African-American musics. (Unpublished doctoral dissertation). University of California, Berkeley.

Jackson, I. (ed.) (1985). *More than drumming: Essays on African and Afro-Latin American music and musicians*. Westport, CT: Greenwood Press.

Japan National Tourism Organization. Shinto Shrines. Retrieved July 15, 2017 from http://www.jnto.go.jp/eng/indepth/cultural/experience/d.html.

Kagan, N. (1995). *Interpersonal Process Recall: Theory and Introduction*, presented by Norman Kagan, in Interpersonal Process Recall 1, Alexandria, VA: Microtraining Associates, 59 mins.

Kalani and Camara, R. (2006). *West-African Drum & Dance: A Yankadi-Macrou Celebration*. Van Nuys CA: Alfred Publishing Company, Inc.

Kouyate, D. (Director). (1994). *Keita!: Heritage of the griot* [Motion picture]. Burkina Faso: California Newsreel.

Lewis, C. (2016). Research Confirms the Health Benefits of Drum Meditation. *Buddhistdoor Global* | 2016-02-18 | Retrieved May 11, 17 from: https://www.buddhistdoor.net/news/research-confirms-the-health-benefits-of-drum-meditation

Lewis, J, Dana, R & Blevins, G (2002). *Substance abuse counseling: An individualized approach*, 3rd ed. Pacific Grove, CA: Brooks/Cole.

Maxfield (1991). Effects of Rhythmic Drumming on EEG and Subjective Experience, as cited in Arrien, A., 1993, *The Four-Fold Way*, San Francisco: Harper Collins.

McBride, R. Retrieved July 17, 2017, from https://mixedblood.info

McCraty R (2017) New Frontiers in Heart Rate Variability and Social Coherence Research: Techniques, Technologies, and Implications for Improving Group Dynamics and Outcomes. *Front. Public Health 5:267. doi: 10.3389/fpubh.2017.00267*

Mews, J. (2014). 5 Main Benefits Of Drumming For Children With Special Needs. *Mewsic Moves*. Retrieved April 21 2017 from https://www.mewsicmoves.com/blog/5-benefits-of-drumming-for-children-with-special-needs

Miller, E.K. and Buschman, T.J. (2013) Brain Rhythms for Cognition and Consciousness. In: *Neurosciences and the Human Person: New Perspectives on Human Activities* A. Battro, S. Dehaene and W. Singer (eds), Pontifical Academy of Sciences, Scripta Varia 121, Vatican City.

Miller, E.K. and Wallis, J.D. (2009) Executive function and higher-order cognition: Definitions and neural substrates. In: *Encyclopedia of Neuroscience, Volume 4*, Squire LR (Ed.), pp 99-104. Oxford: Academic Press.

Native Net. Native American Drums. Retrieved July 15, 2017 from http://www.native-net.org/na/native-american-drums.html.

Newcomb, S. "'Canada' and the 'United States' Are in Turtle Island." Indian Country Today. Retrieved July 22, 2017 from https://indiancountrymedianetwork.com/news/opinions/canada-and-the-united-states-are-in-turtle-island/

Nketia, J.H.K. (2005). *Ethnomusicology and African Music.* Afram Publications: Accra, Ghana.

Oren, A (2008). The use of board games in child psychotherapy. *Journal of Child Psychotherapy.* 38:3, 364-383. DOI: 10.1080/00754170802472893.

Peck, M.S. (1987). *The Different Drum: Community Making and Peace.* New York: Simon & Schuster Inc.

Ponterotto, J. G., & Pedersen, P. B. (1993). *Multicultural aspects of counseling series, Vol. 2. Preventing prejudice: A guide for counselors and educators.* Thousand Oaks, CA: Sage Publications.

Putnam, R.D. (2000). *Bowling Alone: The Collapse and Revival of American Community.* New York: Simon & Schuster.

Rosenbaum, D. (2014) *It's a Jungle In There: How competition and cooperation in the brain shape the mind.* Oxford University Press.

Sacks, O. (2007). *Musicophilia.* New York: Vintage Books.

Smith C[1], Viljoen JT, McGeachie L. (2014). African drumming: a holistic approach to reducing stress and improving health? J Cardiovasc Med (Hagerstown). 2014 Jun;15(6):441-6. doi: 10.2459/JCM.0000000000000046.

Stephenson, J. (2017) Fight Facism with a Dance Party. *Yes Magazine,* posted Aug 11, 2017 Retrieved September 29, 2017 from: http://www.yesmagazine.org/people-power/fight-fascism-with-a-dance-party-20170811.

Stevens, C. (2003). *The Art and Heart of Drum Circles.* Milwaukee WI: Hal Leonard Corporation.

Stevens, P. & Smith, R. (2009). *Substance abuse counseling theory and practice*, 4th ed. Pearson: Saddle River NJ.

Streng, I. (2008). Using therapeutic board games to promote child mental health. *Journal of Public Mental Health*. Vol 7, issue 4, pp 4-16.

Substance abuse treatment admissions of older adults more than doubled from 1992 to 2008 (September 9, 2010). SAMHSA Press Release. Retrieved December 9, 2017, from:
https://www.samhsa.gov/newsroom/press-announcements/201009091100

Sullivan, P. and Blacker, M. (2017). The Effect of Different Phases of Synchrony on Pain Threshold in a Drumming Task. *Frontiers in Psychology*. 8:1034.
doi: 10.3389/fpsyg.2017.01034

Tannen, D. (1990). *You Just Don't Understand: Women and men in conversation.* London: Virago.
Tannen, D. and Bly, R. (1992). *Men and Women: Talking Together* [sound recording]. New York: Sound Horizons Audio-Video, 1992.

Vygotsky, L., edited by Cole, M., John-Steiner, V., Scribner, V., & Souberman, E. (1978). *Mind in Society: The development of higher psychological processes.* Cambridge, MA: Harvard University Press.

Wadaiko Tokara. What is taiko? Retrieved July 15, 2017 from http://www.tokara.net/tokarataiko.html.

Williams, B. M. (2001) *Babatunde Olatunji.* Hall of Fame, Percussive Arts Society [on line]. Retrieved April 17, 2013 from http://www.pas.org/experience/halloffame/OlatunjiBabatunde.aspx

Wilson, E.O. (1975). Man: From Sociobiology to Sociology (Territoriality and Tribalism). In: *Sociobiology - The New Synthesis* pp.547-576. The Belknap Press of Harvard University Press.

Wilson, S. G. (1992). *The drummer's path: Moving the spirit with ritual and traditional drumming.* Vermont: Destiny Books.

Winerman, L. (2012) Neuroplasticity. *APA Monitor*, September 2012, Vol 43, No. 8 p 30.

Wishart, D. (ed.) Sun Dance. Encyclopedia of the Great Plains. Retrieved July 22, 2017 from http://plainshumanities.unl.edu/encyclopedia/doc/egp.rel.046

Zhao, DJ (2014). No drums allowed: Afro rhythmic mutations in America. *This is Africa*. August 1, 2014. Retrived March 18, 2018, from

https://thisisafrica.me/lifestyle/drums-allowed-afro-rhythmic-mutations-america/

About the Author

Signe M. Kastberg has been a counselor educator and psychotherapist for over 20 years. She completed her doctoral degree in Human Development at the University of Rochester (NY), the Ed.M. degree at Harvard University, and a Fulbright Scholarship for independent research in Copenhagen, Denmark. She also worked as a Continuing Education director for over a decade.

Dr. Kastberg first discovered her affinity for African drumming in Ithaca, New York, and has benefited from many teachers (and students, and dancers) in developing a feel for the polyrhythms of West Africa in particular. Her interests in traditional West-African drumming also led to the study of other cultural contexts for drumming. She participated in Taiko drumming class, and built her own Native American buffalo drum to participate in sacred ceremony under the guidance of a Native elder.

As the current book details, Dr. Kastberg has applied her knowledge about health aspects of drumming, combined with the rich history of drumming in Africa, to teach clients in a variety of settings how to use drumming therapeutically. The path to healing can take many forms.

Dr. Kastberg is also author of numerous book chapters and articles on topics relevant to counseling, psychotherapy, and human development. In 2007 she published, *Servants in the House of the Masters: A Social Class Primer for Educators, Helping Professionals, and Others Who Want to Change the World.* This book is based on her dissertation research and subsequent interactive speaking engagements around the country.

To provide feedback on the current book, or to arrange speaking engagements, contact signe.jag@gmail.com.